Is the Health Service for Healing?

First published in 2006 by
Liberties Press
Guinness Enterprise Centre | Taylor's Lane | Dublin 8 | Ireland
www. LibertiesPress .com | info@libertiespress.com
Editorial: +353 (1) 402 0805 | sean@libertiespress.com
Sales and marketing: +353 (1) 415 1224 | peter@libertiespress.com

Trade enquiries to CMD Distribution
55A Spruce Avenue | Stillorgan Industrial Park | Blackrock | County Dublin
Tel: +353 (1) 294 2560
Fax: +353 (1) 294 2564

Copyright © Risteárd Mulcahy, 2006

The author has asserted his moral rights.

ISBN-10: 1–905483–15–5
ISBN-13: 978–1–905483–15–0

2 4 6 8 10 9 7 5 3 1

A CIP record for this title is available from the British Library

Cover design by Ros Murphy
Set in Garamond

Printed in Ireland by Colour Books
Unit 105 | Baldoyle Industrial Estate | Dublin 13

Liberties Press is a member of Clé, the Irish Book Publishers' Association

This book is sold subject to the condition that it shall not, by way of trade or otherwise, be lent, resold, hired out or otherwise circulated, without the publisher's prior consent, in any form other than that in which it is published and without a similar condition including this condition being imposed on the subsequent publisher.

No part of this publication may be reproduced or transmitted in any form or by any means, electronic or mechanical, including photocopying, recording or storage in any information or retrieval system, without the prior permission of the publisher in writing.

Is the Health Service for Healing?

A Doctor's Defence of
Medicine's Samaritan Role

Risteárd Mulcahy

PRIMUM NON NOCERE

Contents

	Acknowledgements	7
	Foreword by Prof. Niall O'Higgins	9
	Introduction	13
1	The Question of Equity	28
2	Private Hospitals and Public Welfare	37
3	The Medical Profession	54
4	The Nursing Profession	74
5	The Role of Government	78
6	Health Promotion	86
	References	93
	Glossary of Medical Terms	96

Acknowledgements

I am grateful to many people who assisted me in completing this monograph. I must of course confirm that all the views expressed in the text are mine. While on many issues I found agreement, it is clear that other opinions prevailed. The health service in Ireland is not without its contentious aspects.

I would like to mention the following, who were helpful in providing material or in responding to certain questions: Niall O'Higgins, Nicky Jermyn, Brendan Drumm, Séamus Healy, Mary Harney TD, Liam Twomey TD, Liz McManus TD, John Gormley TD, Vincent Sheridan, Bernadette Carr, Jimmie Sheehan, Pat Lyons, Mark Redmond, Michael Cullen, Fintan O'Toole, Maev-Ann Wren, Ian Graham, Cecily Kelleher, Leslie Daly, Miriam Wiley, John Barton, Dermot Hourihane, and Richard and Hugh Mulcahy. Ulick O'Connor provided encouragement, and Oliver McCullen read the text with an eagle's eye.

I am grateful to the staff of the Central Statistics Office, to the staff of the ESRI and to the medical librarians at St Vincent's and UCD, Earlsfort Terrace, for their courtesy and willing cooperation over many years. I am grateful to the editors of *Medicine Weekly*, the *Irish Medical News* and the *Irish Medical Times*. Without their reporting of current medical affairs, I could not have found and sourced much of the information in the text.

I was inspired by Dr Emer Shelley's great knowledge of the Irish medical scene. She helped as best she could to keep me within the bounds of common sense. I have already thanked my wife, Louise, for her patience and forbearance, and for sharing her knowledge of nursing and of hospital organisation in Ireland.

As always, I owe a lot to my publisher, Seán O'Keeffe of Liberties Press, for his careful editing and his close interest in the subject of the monograph.

Foreword

In peacetime it would be expected that democratic countries would place education, health and social welfare as the leading priorities for government. When a stable political system and economic affluence are added, society expects coherent and fair systems in areas of such cardinal importance. That grave inequalities are widespread and deep in the health services in Ireland should be of concern and should not be accepted.

Much time and expense has been given to the establishment of task forces, working groups and committees charged with the preparation of recommendations and guidelines upon which public-health policy can be based. Many documents and publications are developed, acknowledged and approved by government but, sadly, action and implementation are frequently postponed or avoided. Frustration follows inevitably.

In *Is the Health Service for Healing*, Prof. Risteárd Mulcahy draws attention to many of the inequalities in the Irish health system, particularly those of access to primary and specialist medical services for non-emergency care, the hospital-beds crisis, waiting lists for medical and surgical procedures, and the lack of facilities for people with chronic illness. He analyses the derivation and details of current difficulties, attributing many of the problems and their causes to lack of strategic leadership by government, piecemeal or ad hoc arrangements, and expedient policies that are intrinsically unsound. He proposes, as he did as far back as 1959, that health issues be removed from the Department of Health to a semi-autonomous body, dissociated from party politics, made up of representation from all relevant interests and reporting only to the Department of Finance.

To quote the physician and medical educationalist Sir Cyril Chantler, 'Medicine used to be simple, ineffective and relatively safe. Now it is complex, effective and potentially dangerous.' No society, however wealthy, can afford the indiscriminate use of technology that is currently available in medicine. Prof. Mulcahy is sharply critical of the way in which huge commercial pressures now drive the practice of medicine and are displacing, even replacing, the clinical skills required and expected of doctors. This trend has obvious implications for the education and training of doctors, and the reduction of the time available to medical students for contact with patients is another target for criticism. In the same broad context, the removal of the nursing schools from their central location within the hospitals has reduced the motivation, spirit and commitment of nurses to direct hands-on patient care. Perhaps instead of moving nursing schools to the university, educational authorities should have moved the university to the nursing schools in the hospital setting.

Prof. Mulcahy also blames the medical profession and the professional training bodies for their failure to speak clearly in defence of the ethical principles upon which medical practice is founded, and for what he perceives as a reluctance on the part of the profession to embrace the idea and the practice of audit, although he acknowledges that the surgical community has been encouraging and requesting accurate clinical (and administrative) audit since 1980 on the grounds that audit is a powerful tool for improving standards and is not primarily intended as a mechanism to censure individuals. BreastCheck, the national breast cancer screening programme, is an excellent example of what can be achieved when clinical and administrative expertise is combined with rigorous audit. The quality of this programme is at least as good as any in the world.

He aims his most powerful arrows at the proliferation of for-profit private hospitals, devoting a full section of the book to the dangers of privatisation in terms of patient care and the financial cost. He strongly opposes the application of for-profit hospitals as part of government policy for Ireland and draws attention to the likely misuses and overspending which he considers to be necessarily associated with this arrangement. Furthermore, he believes that doctors who are involved as medical consultants in profit-making hospitals and who are at the same time shareholders in these institutions inevitably have a conflict of interest that is 'unacceptable to the profession and disturbing to the public'.

The monograph is not a mere chronicle of issues but a clearly expressed analytical treatise, written in unambiguous style and with surgical precision. Prof. Mulcahy is never strident or doctrinaire. He may see only part of the multiplicity of aspects on some issues and may sometimes draw conclusions that are incomplete, but he is always fair. His treatise adds to the robust debate currently swirling around the health services in Ireland. It is therefore a welcome and timely document.

Prof. Mulcahy's critique draws on his long-committed personal experience as a clinical specialist who was also involved in medical politics. He has had a lifelong concern for the health of society in general as well as for the welfare of individual patients under his care. His devotion to his society is unquestioned, and his scholarship is acknowledged. His career and writings have been devoid of any self-interest, and his analytical mind has allowed him, in Newman's words, 'to develop a clear, conscious view of his own opinions and judgements, a truth in developing them, an eloquence in expressing them and a force in urging them . . . an ability to see things as they are, to go right to the point, to disentangle a skein of thought, to detect what is sophistical and to discard what is irrelevant'. Risteárd Mulcahy and John Henry Newman, had they met, might well have 'tired the sun with talking and sent him down the sky'.

Niall O'Higgins
November 2006

INTRODUCTION

In writing this monograph, I am aware that I am entering the minefield of health-service politics and policies. Retired from hospital practice for nearly eighteen years, and long since out of the corridors of power, I am not competent to write an account of the complexities of our health service, nor am I in a position to do extensive research on the subject. This has to be left to more competent authors, such as Ruth Barrington, who provided a history of the service from 1900 to 1970,[1] and A. Dale Tussing and Maev-Ann Wren, who have recently published a detailed and critical account of the current situation.[2] That the health services in Ireland have not been neglected by writers, economists, sociologists and commissions is clear from the thirty-nine reports on the subject issued since 2000, which are referenced by Tussing and Wren.

My purpose therefore is not to provide a broad examination of the health service but to deal with certain aspects which need attention if we are to design for this country a health service which will serve the interests of patients, the ethical standards of the medical professions, and the country's professional and financial needs. The issues I raise are pertinent to my own career as a physician and cardiologist from 1950 to 1988 and reflect my long-standing interest in our health service over this period.

*

The health service appears to be in constant ferment. Responsibility for its failings must be shared at least to some degree by all those concerned with its organisation. This is clear in the current culture of blame and conflict, where no consensus on aspects of policy, however fundamental, can be reached. In looking at health-delivery problems dispassionately, I appreciate that my views will ruffle the feathers of some of my colleagues in the field of medicine as well as other health professionals, administrators and politicians. We cannot find a satisfactory and equitable long-term solution to the country's health-care problems unless all elements concerned are consulted, willing to compromise and prepared to seek common ground.

Although retired from hospital practice for eighteen years, I have kept close to the medical scene as director of the exercise stress testing facility at the Charlemont Clinic in Dublin. I act on behalf of colleagues in the clinic and on behalf of outside physicians and general practitioners. In this capacity I have had access to many patients' medical histories and their experience of the medical services, both in general practice and in the private and public hospital services.

The central health authorities have been proceeding with policies which may appear expedient in solving current difficulties in the health service but will almost certainly lead to serious problems in the long term. Minister Harney and her officials are not sufficiently aware of the views of health professionals about her policies, apart perhaps from those of our trade-union organisations. She is proceeding too rashly with expedient but impractical solutions without seeking the views of our academic and educational organisations, or of individual doctors, nurses and other health professionals; it is these people, more than others, who can provide useful views about health matters. She seems to be quite unaware of the adverse effects her privatisation proposals will have on the ethical standards of our profession.

It is remarkable that the present government is undertaking a major initiative in relation to our future health services without seeking a wider view from parliament and the people, and by ignoring many recommendations relating to health strategy by experts in the field. Surely the future of our health service merits more consideration from parliament, particularly as future health care and social needs in all countries are facing a looming crisis because of cost, the question of equity, rapid demographic changes, the increasing commercialisation of medicine, high-tech medical advances, litigation and, most important, the weakening of vocationalism and of professional and public ethics. I fear particularly for the ethos and ethical standards of my profession, where patient care was the only consideration of doctors and other health professionals in the past. If we fail in our ethical standards, it is the patient and the public who must pay the price.

We cannot ignore the serious influence that with-profit private hospitals may have on the cost of providing health services and on ethical standards of the medical profession. Before the surge of with-profit hospitals in Ireland and the increasing commercialisation of life under the Celtic Tiger, we doctors were privileged to have access to our patients without any financial influence which might militate against our total commitment to patient care. In April 2006, Ms Harney, in defending her support for the privatisation of health care, pleaded that such privatisation was part of recent health care policies not only in America but also in Canada and many European countries. I am aware that this is so, but one must dispute her contention that the widespread privatisation in other countries justifies our following in the same direction. Many of these countries are facing the same problems of cost, and I do not think that their problems will be solved by private investors. The wider adoption of private medicine and the recourse to private investment is a reaction to the frustrations caused by the burgeoning cost of medical care and the failure to adapt health management to changing times. It is perhaps an act of desperation on the part of the central cost providers.

Increasing cost, and a deterioration of professional ethics, are inseparable from privatisation, where the profit motive for investors becomes the driving force of the institution. In many countries, including Ireland, the commercialisation and privatisation of health care is simply an attractive expedient to shore up a service which is getting out of control in terms of cost and poor management. In short, profit-driven privatisation can only aggravate the cost problem. It is also likely that, as medical practice becomes more commercialised, the public will respond by being less solicitous of our professional standing and more likely to have recourse to litigation. In the May and June 1959 issues of the Fine Gael monthly journal of current affairs the *National Observer*, I wrote two articles about the problems of the health services in Ireland, and the possible solutions to such problems. In view of the setting up of the Health Service Executive (HSE) in 2004 by Mary Harney, it is appropriate to record my views of almost half a century ago:

I am sure that the first important step is that health administration should be removed from the milieu of party politics. This can only be achieved by transferring the main responsibility for affairs of health from the Department of Health to an authority constituted along the same lines as our semi-state or semi-autonomous bodies, such as the electricity, turf and transport concerns. I believe that this change would enormously simplify administration in the future whilst providing a continuity of policy in health legislation which is badly needed and which would be appreciated by all people interested in social welfare.

This independent health body should be established with strong and comprehensive executive powers over all health services in the country that require the assistance of public money. It should also bear the responsibility for the direction of new health policy. It should be answerable to the government on matters of finance.

I suggested that this body should have full representation from the medical profession as well as from other health professionals and from administration. My contention was that, in 1959, the health service was weighed down with anomalies and inefficiencies, that it lacked a coordinated focus, that its shortcomings were aggravated by political influences at central and local levels, that the department and local health authorities shared much of the blame for this situation, and that the views of the medical profession were ignored in relation to policy and performance. My one hopeful comment referred to the success of the Voluntary Health Insurance Board (VHI), which had been established three years earlier.

During visits to cardiac-research centres in the United States in 1971, I studied some aspects of the American health system. I was

INTRODUCTION

particularly interested in the Kaiser Permanente programme, which has its headquarters in Oakland in California and centres in a few contiguous states. It was established as a pre-payment group-practice service and is described as such on the Kaiser Permanente website:

> Kaiser Permanente is America's leading integrated health plan. Founded in 1945, it is a pre-payment program with headquarters in Oakland, California. Kaiser Permanente serves the health-care needs of about 8.2 million members in nine states and the District of Columbia. Today it encompasses the not-for-profit Kaiser Foundation Health Plan, Inc., Kaiser Foundation Hospitals and their subsidiaries, and the for-profit Permanente Medical Groups. Nationwide, Kaiser Permanente includes approximately 136,000 technical, administrative and clerical employees and over 11,000 physicians representing all specialties.

The Kaiser Permanente Health Care Plan is a non-profit system which might have some relevance to our current planning. It should be studied by those who are determining future health policy, and particularly those who favour compulsory or voluntary health insurance. The VHI might possibly adopt the Kaiser Permanente system by widening its interest in the provision of health care. When I first visited the KP headquarters in 1971, it had about 2 million subscribers and two thousand physicians. It appears to have prospered since then and now includes disadvantaged and chronically ill patients, as in all national health systems. The associated for-profit Permanente Medical Groups refer to the physicians who are salaried by Kaiser Permanente. KP provides incentives to their physicians and surgeons to earn more by avoiding unnecessary hospital admissions and by discouraging over-investigation and over-treatment of patients.

In 1971, when I was in Oakland, KP required 1.7 beds per thousand members, compared to a national average in the United States of 3.7 beds. Hospital stays were also shorter and, significantly, in the latest report on their website the group requires two-thirds fewer hospital beds than the American average. The publication by Feachem and colleagues, in which comparisons are made between

Kaiser Permanente and the British National Health Service, is necessary reading.[3] Cost is about the same per patient, but the efficiency of KP is much greater. Research into health services is a strong component of KP's programme and must contribute to its high standards of efficiency. We have had our own well-researched reports, but these have failed to evoke the interest and the policies of our politicians. Efficiency in planning and administration, and a medical profession with disincentives to admit patients to hospital and to avoid over-treatment and the excessive use of tests, can provide a system which can cope with the needs of modern medical practice within reasonable financial bounds.

The incentives aimed at controlling excessive admissions and investigations at KP are based on a system whereby physicians and surgeons share the money which remains after the expenses of the system are paid, thus adding to their fixed salaries. As a unique health insurance system, Kaiser Permanente may not be suitable as a national system for Ireland, but I mention it because it differs fundamentally from the approach in the hospital culture here, where doctors and hospitals have a strong incentive, for a variety of reasons, to admit patients to hospital, thus adding to the cost and complexity of health care. The medical profession attached to the KP service has a strong tradition of audit and peer review. Informal discussions about the system among colleagues when I returned to Ireland in 1971 elicited some interest but no action. A thirty-page review I subsequently wrote on the American and Irish health care systems remains unpublished.

At a later date, in 1974, after I had retired as president of the Irish Medical Association, I was to chair the IMA working party which recommended the adoption of a one-tier nationwide hospital compulsory health insurance system, using the Voluntary Health Insurance as a model.[4] This policy was adopted by the Central Council of the IMA, and the report was published, with an added editorial, in the Association's journal. It apparently made no impression on the politicians and the Department of Health. Implementation of the report might have been unrealistic under the economic conditions of the time, but with our current prosperity it would be feasible, equitable, more efficient and certainly more economical than our current drift towards an American solution.

I spent a week recently in Finland with a retired professor of medicine and his family, many of whom were also involved in medicine. The Finns have a single-tier system with little private medicine. It is financed by central funds and provides free services for the entire community. There appears to be general satisfaction with the services there. Before launching us into a costly, divisive, iniquitous and profit-driven system which bears no relation to the services in Northern Ireland, the UK or the Continent, the authorities here should learn from the experience of these countries. Has the current government taken any measures to study the systems in other countries, and have they consulted with those who are at the coalface of the service in Ireland?

Maev-Ann Wren's *Unhealthy State: Anatomy of a Sick Society* was published in June 2003.[5] My monograph is simply an up-to-date extension of a commentary I wrote shortly after the publication of Ms Wren's book. *Unhealthy State* was written at a time of considerable ferment in Ireland in relation to the delivery of the health services. Its examination of the service was detailed, comprehensive and highly critical, as was that of its successor, by Tussing and Wren.[2] It appeared at about the same time as several other reports which had been commissioned to examine different aspects of the service. The earliest of these was the Deloitte and Touche report ordered by the Department of Health to examine the value for money offered by the service. The Prospectus report (to assess functions and structures of the service) appeared in 2003, and the Hanly report (on medical staffing) was published in early 2004. They were also commissioned by the Department of Health. The Brennan report (management and control of spending) was commissioned by the Department of Finance.

Many of the recommendations of the Prospectus and Brennan reports have been implemented, including the setting up of the Health Service Executive (HSE) and some improvement in community services. One wonders how much the other reports cost in terms of money and the input of experts, and to what degree their combined influence added to the solution of our health-service problems as proposed by Ms Harney.

Unhealthy State understandably provoked a reaction among the medical professions, the public and politicians. Wren was particularly critical of the lack of equity in the service, with poor access to primary care for the less privileged members of the community. She attributed many of the problems within the service to under-funding of health by successive governments. She was critical of the consultants in the public hospitals because of their method of payment, their high average income in the public service, and the high income of some who are in private practice. She was also critical of the existing mix of public and private medicine, and of the fees charged by general practitioners.

Ms Wren underlined the fact that the Irish health service has evolved over the years in a piecemeal and haphazard fashion because of poor long-term central policy and strategy. She drew particular attention to a failure to face up to abuses which she attributes to the medical profession, local politicians and other some dissident groups. She was particularly critical of the recent Fianna Fáil administrations. The reports which have been issued on health affairs, widely quoted in her pages, and her detailed analysis, led to extensive comment in the popular and medical press. The media comments were generally critical of the government and the medical profession, while the medical press generally sought to defend the consultants and the medical profession.

The Brennan report was critical of the role of the consultants, and raised the hackles of the Irish Hospital Consultants' Association (IHCA). As regards the Hanly report, dissenting groups among the public and even among doctors have been critical of its recommendations because of the perceived demotion of some of the provincial hospitals. There is no evidence that any government since the creation of the Department of Health in 1944 has attempted to propose a fully integrated and comprehensive health service, with the possible exception of the Public Health Bill of 1944 during the Fianna Fáil administration of the time. The authorities have generally been satisfied with the two-tier system based on public hospitals supported by Sweepstake funds and subsequently public funds, and private non-profit hospitals managed by religious and other charitable groups, and supported by the VHI. The rather abrupt departure of the religious from the medical sector in recent years, added to demographic changes, medical advances and professional influences, has destabilised the status quo and left the system with serious problems, which our usual attempts at patching up are unlikely to remedy. Despite numerous valuable reports and enquiries into hospital and health matters, starting with the Fitzgerald report on hospital regionalisation in 1967, most attempts to rationalise the service have led to controversy and muddle, and the failure of government to formulate a proper health structure or to use its authority to deal with minority opinion and disagreements because of local party electoral considerations.

The Tussing and Wren report (2006) was sponsored and published by the Irish Congress of Trade Unions (ICTU), representing the trade unions IMPACT and SIPTU, the Irish Medical Organisation (IMO) and the Irish Nurses' Organisation (INO). It is an important and up-to-date report which is now receiving the same publicity as Wren's original report and which should have been crucial in influencing government intentions if it had become an integral part of ICTU's negotiations with government. I was assured by a spokesman of ICTU that the question of equity and of the cost and ethical implications of the authority's action in encouraging investment-led privatisation are an important part of the unions' remit.

The recent agreement reached by ICTU and the government did not, however, refer to health-service matters although it did include some social issues. Since then, an ICTU spokesman informs me that ICTU's objections to the investment in private hospitals through tax incentives will be raised at a conference in autumn 2006. But Ms Harney's plans are proceeding inexorably at the moment, and they have already raised considerable interest among private investors and financial institutions. If ICTU are opposed to Ms Harney's privatisation policies, they should say so in public now, thus supporting Tussing and Wren and those of us who oppose the privatisation route. Tussing and Wren's book, the product of a year's intensive research by two authorities on the subject, is a most important and cogent analysis of our health-delivery problems and a constructive contribution to the solution of these problems. ICTU sponsored their report; do they support the report's findings? The heads of the IMO and the INO have spoken out against with-profit private hospitals. Are their views personal, or are they speaking on behalf of their members?

What are the basic elements of an ideal health-delivery service which might exist within the many political, financial, professional, social and cultural restraints that exist? That such a system has not been devised in Western countries is clearly apparent. It is inevitable that the rapid advances in medical care and technology that have been made since the mid-twentieth century, together with an increasingly assertive, demanding, litigious and educated public, an ageing population, and the gradual erosion of the extended family, are presenting health authorities with serious challenges. Add to these the incentives that doctors in Ireland have to admit patients to hospital for investigation and treatment rather than to deal with them at outpatient level, the unique consultant contract, the departure of the religious as owners of public and non-profit private hospitals, and burgeoning immigration, which is swelling the numbers requiring health care.

The ideal system must include immediate access to primary and specialist care for the entire community; efficient central direction and effective administration at local level; well-trained health professionals; emphasis on cost efficiency as well as high professional standards through audit and peer review; and financial investment which must have some limits and which is commensurate with other demands on the public and private purses. Finally, there must be personal responsibility among the public in utilising the service.

The one-tier systems that exist in the Scandinavian countries, in Finland, in Switzerland and in Israel appear to be the most satisfactory in terms of public satisfaction and affordability. These are economies where long-term socialist policies have led to high taxation, particularly of the rich, and to minimal divisions on lines of social class. It seems that the definitions of public and private may be irrelevant when we are proposing a one-tier system. The systems in Switzerland and Israel are based on compulsory health insurance;

like the VHI in Ireland, different premiums are designed to provide different services, but basic health needs are available to everybody, and without long waiting lists. Because of the lack of a structured health strategy in solving the problems of the health service here in Ireland, it seems essential that the different European systems should be researched to determine the likely best system for this country.

I am not competent to deal with the matter of the cost of the health services. Cost is influenced by a bewildering variety of factors – social, demographic, technical, professional, administrative, managerial and financial – and comparing the current and future cost of different systems in different countries is a complex task. The reader seeking information on cost and system comparisons should refer to Chapter 2 of the Tussing/Wren report. Barrett and Bergin[6] have estimated the cost of the Irish system up to 2050, but their estimate of future cost, and other prospective estimates in the UK and elsewhere, may prove to be very wide of the mark, bearing in mind the many variables which influence the cost of health care and the many uncertainties which we and future generations face on this fragile planet.

Table 1 (on page 24) provides the GDP levels for the fifteen European countries in 2003 (OECD Health Data, 2005). The cost of the Irish 'system' has risen dramatically during the last five years, but it started at a very low base five years ago. It is now likely to be above the European average. Our costs have probably continued to rise since the latest data were published, but this does not necessarily correspond to a commensurate improvement in the health service.

We need to understand the high cost and unsatisfactory features of the American system. The huge cost of health care in the United States, at more than 15 percent of GDP, contrasts starkly with that of other European countries. A recent publication from the US government projects that expenditure on health will continue to rise in the next ten years and will reach 20 percent of the economy, or one of every five dollars spent by the end of that period. It had already reached $1.9 trillion in 2004.[7] If our health service follows

TABLE 1: Total health expenditure as percentage of GDP in 2003 in fifteen European countries

	2003	RANKING
Germany	11.1	1
France	10.1	2
Greece	9.9	3
Nethrelands	9.8	4
Belgium	9.6	5
Portugal	9.6	6
Sweden	9.4	7
Denmark	9.0	8
Ireland*	8.9	9
Italy	8.4	10
Spain	7.7	11
Austria	7.5	12
Finland	7.4	13
Luxembourg	6.9	14
United Kingdom**	n/a	
EU average	9.0	

* Irish data as percent of GNP; GNP is used as a measure of national income because GDP includes multinationals' repatriated profits and is an overestimation.

** UK 7.7 percent in 2002

the American model, as seems likely under Mary Harney, our spending is likely to rocket from its 2003 level of 8.9 percent to close to or higher than the American level.

Figure 1 (on page 25) confirms that there is some correlation between health expenditure and life expectancy in thirty chosen countries, but the correlation is weak. There are other confounding factors which influence life expectancy, but many recent publications confirm that primary prevention through population lifestyle changes plays a dominant part in the recent improvement of life expectancy in the Western World. There is no strong relationship between money spent on interventional medicine, the general health of the population, and life expectancy. Nor does money

FIGURE 1: Scattergram showing correlation between life expectancy and spending on health in thirty countries

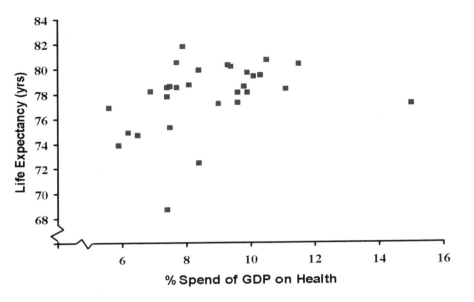

necessarily equate with efficiency and cost efficacy, as is clear from poor American experience and the exemplary record of the Kaiser Permanente Group.

The VHI premiums have increased by 98 percent over the last eight years and are predicted to increase another 50 percent by 2009.[8] The premiums will rise by 12 percent in 2006, as they did in 2005. According to the VHI authorities, these substantial increases will occur even if the risk-equalisation case is settled in VHI's favour. In a recent publication, Vincent Sheridan, the CEO of the VHI, stated that private health insurance is close to saturation point.[9]

With the escalating costs of medical care, it would be wise to assume that these increases, at three to four times the rise in the cost-of-living index, are likely to continue as a result of, and may even be accentuated by, Mary Harney's intention to build eleven with-profit hospitals. In fact, the burgeoning developments in high-tech diagnostic and treatment methods, and the gradual decline of clinical medicine, can only add further to the cost of health care. Future costs may make it impossible to satisfy both a demanding public and a profession which places patient care before cost and which must face the reality of the gradual reduction in cost efficacy of medical treatment in terms of morbidity and lives saved. It is inevitable that cost control will need to be applied to medical services, whether private or public, including such controversial issues as cosmetic surgery.

It might well be asked if it is possible to provide a service which would satisfy everybody, bearing in mind the increasing cost of medical technology, and the prospect of a more demanding and ageing society, where the old are subjected to expensive 'salvage' medicine – something which itself raises serious ethical and financial questions. Before dealing with specific aspects of the health services, the following summary lists some of the main points which might be considered in seeking the best solution to our needs:

- § A compulsory health-insurance system for the entire population.
- § Such a system should be under the control of a non-governmental agency with full representation from all relevant interests. It should be answerable to the Department of Finance.
- § The service should be financed by central funds, health insurance companies and/or government bonds with reasonably attractive fixed dividends. With-profit investment allowing substantial tax incentives should be prohibited.
- § Independent private hospitals should be allowed only with the approval of the central health authority and the health insurers.
- § Equal access to primary care should be available to all citizens.
- § The service should be progressive in providing up-to-date clinical and technical facilities.
- § Apart from clear medical indications, all incentives to admit patients to hospital should be eliminated from the system.
- § A careful examination of bed needs in our principal hospitals should be carried out before decisions are made about our exact bed requirements.

- § Regional hospital groups should be formed, each group with a single board of management.
- § Hospital consultants should be organised in a hierarchical manner to ensure maximum efficiency. The medical chief of the consultant staff should have equal status with the lay CEO.
- § A compulsory and effective audit within the profession aimed at controlling the burgeoning drug and intervention culture which is a feature of Western society.
- § A substantial increase in community investment to care for the chronic sick, the old and the disabled, and particularly to encourage home care where feasible. This should precede any major increase in hospital beds.
- § A change of culture, encouraged by public education, requiring a greater sense of responsibility for one's own health and that of one's dependants.
- § Overuse of the service by the public might be partly controlled by charging a proportion of the cost of health care to the patient.
- § Medical education and practice to adopt a more equal balance between a drug/intervention culture and a culture emphasising personal responsibility for health.
- § Political action to encourage aerobic activity at a personal rather than an elitist level, to encourage health and general education, and to implement appropriate political and legal reform. To achieve a healthier society, education is more important than the provision of optimum elective health services.

In commenting three years ago on Ms Wren's book, I dealt with the following subjects raised by her: the question of equity, the public/private mix, the role of the medical profession, the role of the nursing profession, the role of government and, finally, the poor relation of the service, health promotion. Some of my comments are based on the assumption that we continue with the current two-tier system of separate public and private practice, a system which appears to me to be inconsistent with the mores of a modern, democratic, prosperous and rational state but morally acceptable if the with-profit element is discarded.

1

The Question of Equity

Inequity in education and social justice breeds ill health, as is evident among the poor, the unemployed, prisoners, and those who live in a poor environment. (Realistically, we should be more concerned about better education for the masses rather than a better health service.) Inequalities in access to optimum services are perhaps the most glaring shortcoming in the current health service. Fortunately, this problem does not exist to the same extent for patients who are acutely ill and who require emergency attention. Inequality exists for non-acute patients at both primary general-practitioner and hospital levels. To achieve equity would require drastic changes and more assertive authority by government.

Equity at a primary level could be more closely achieved by increasing the number of doctor-only medical cards to a higher threshold of income and by including others who may be disadvantaged for one reason or another. A substantial number of those who are currently disadvantaged by the lack of a medical card will clearly be assisted by the recently introduced doctor-only card (although it seems that there has not been a great response among those qualified to receive them – evidence no doubt of the high disposable incomes of many people in Ireland today, as well as of the delay in processing applications). The threshold of eligibility has been increased recently, bringing us easier access to GP care for the entire population. If we retain a two-tier system in Ireland, the doctor-only card may alleviate current hardship in relation to general practice, particularly with the added schemes to reduce the direct cost of medications. The alternative to the current proposals is to introduce a free GP service based on compulsory health insurance. It is not always easy to find one's general practitioner at short notice nowadays, but current moves to establish GP co-ops and GP groups attached to hospitals may greatly improve the efficiency of primary care.

There are serious inequities in the elective hospital services, where public patients are subjected to unacceptably long waiting lists for specialist consultations and treatment in hospital. They are also subjected to other disadvantages, including less certain contact with consultants, and more dependence on doctors in training in their management and treatment, not to mention the cancellation of appointments and services, including operations, because of shortages of beds and staff, and other shortcomings.

The National Treatment Purchase Fund (NTPF) has been in operation since 2002. It is an impractical and costly answer to the long-term needs of our public system. Its cost implications are particularly evident from the fact that many patients benefiting by the scheme are admitted following the allotted delay to the same hospital where they have been on the waiting list – surely an anomaly that raises questions about the NTPF as a practical solution. It also raises the point that the consultants may be partly responsible for the long waiting lists if they can deal more expeditiously with the private patient under the same circumstances as the public patient. Has the minister or the NTPF authorities expressed a view about this anomaly?

Of 10,500 patients who were offered outpatient appointments under the NTPF, only 3,310 accepted. Investigations were scheduled for 585 of these, and 1,845 required surgery. The rest were discharged to their GP or moved to a referring hospital.[10] Three thousand three hundred of the 10,500 patients did not attend because they had already been removed from the waiting list, underlining the need to investigate the real nature of waiting lists. Is the NTPF part of a serious health strategy or is it simply another knee-jerk expedient in response to current health demands?

Shortage of beds and shortage of staff are considered to be

major factors in the creation of long waiting lists. Prof. Brendan Drumm, director of the Health Services Executive (HSE), is probably correct in stating that increasing the number of hospital beds is not the primary answer to solving the pressure on Accident and Emergency (A&E) departments and the bed shortage. (He adds a caveat about the need for more beds with a likely population increase through immigration.) It is likely that some increase in public hospital beds may ease the current situation and that other problems might be alleviated by providing more money and other inducements to attract suitable professional staff and to provide better rostering services. More efficient use of beds might be more effective and less costly. If GPs and consultants had no incentive to admit patients to hospital, it is possible that we might not need to increase the number of beds, although the effect of current heavy immigration on bed needs is an additional factor. We have evidence from abroad, such as from the Kaiser Permanente system, and even from some of our own hospitals, where the standards of management are high and where the consultants play a significant part in planning and in administration, that the provision of more beds is not necessarily the answer. A study by the ESRI questioned the efficiency of bed management, particularly in the smaller hospitals.[11] The report states that there were often huge differences across hospitals in relation to efficiency in terms of occupancy rates and duration of stay.

A number of beds in our hospitals are currently occupied by patients who cannot be discharged because of the poor community facilities to care for the old, the permanently disabled and those in unsuitable domestic circumstances. More beds and better facilities for the old, the infirm and the chronically ill should be found in suitable primary institutions as part of our social services and in order to alleviate the pressure on our more expensive secondary and tertiary hospitals.

There is a strong incentive for the profession to admit patients to hospital rather than deal with them at outpatient level. The health-insurance companies pay more to doctors and hospitals for in-patient rather than outpatient care. Outpatient services are often overcrowded and may not be well organised for planning and carrying out necessary investigations. No hostels are available for patients and relatives requiring overnight stays, and admission for investigation suits the busy doctor, where the investigation may be arranged by in-patient staff. While the insurance agencies take some steps to prevent unnecessary admissions, such an admission may suit the doctor financially, and it may also suit the patient because of the better insurance support for in-patient treatment. Fear of litigation may also influence a tendency to admit patients on inadequate clinical grounds.

We should give priority to the provision of much better facilities in terms of community care at domestic and institutional levels, and of hospice care. This proposal is also close to the top of Prof. Drumm's thinking. The Health Service Executive (HSE) has announced its intention to carry out an assessment of the long-term needs of older people, and the Cabinet is seeking a means of funding such an initiative.[12] We must anticipate the inevitable increase in the proportion of older people during future decades, and the prolongation of life among the terminally ill – a circumstance which Illich describes as the prolongation of death. The increasing use of day care or overnight care should be further encouraged, and a reduction in inappropriate admissions should result from efficient triage services and the presence of more senior medical personnel in accident-and-emergency departments. Better facilities for outpatient investigation and treatment in our hospitals would contribute to a lower admission rate. The availability of suitable hostel facilities for patients and relatives close to hospitals seems a sensible and economical means of reducing bed occupancy.

Every effort should be made, both at insurance and professional levels, to eliminate the incentive to admit patients to hospital. Clearly a more accessible GP service would reduce A&E attendances, as might a more realistic legal and cultural approach to the problems of binge-drinking in the community.

A policy simply devoted to increasing the number of beds and providing more money for the health service would not of itself solve the problems of service and cost. Without tackling the problem of inappropriate in-patient admission, the incentives to admit patients, and the reduction in the average stay of patients, hospital reform would be difficult. We need improved staffing levels, particularly among nurses and consultants, and a reduction in the non-consultant/consultant ratio if we are to find a satisfactory new consultant contract. There should be full overview of investigations and treatment ordered by non-consultant junior colleagues. A reduction in the administrator/consultant ratio is feasible if consultants combine their medical duties with a collateral part in administration.

Added to these, a careful analysis of the nature of waiting lists is mandatory. For instance, I believe that the waiting list for heart surgery was long because many of those who are awaiting heart-bypass surgery did not qualify for surgical treatment according to the limited trial indications available to us. Coronary surgery is on the decline and has been overtaken by less invasive angioplasty and much improved medical treatment. We are handicapped in this area because we lack modern trials to inform us about the optimum management of many patients with non-acute coronary disease.[13] Heart surgery and angioplasty may seem more attractive to the patient and doctor because they provide a more compelling and immediate solution than the less dramatic medical intervention based on patient counselling and co-operation, and the highly effective risk-factor modification and drugs available to the present-day cardiologist. I believe that all my cardiological colleagues would say that urgent cases for heart surgery are dealt with promptly, confirming that the public hospitals provide a high standard of service for all acute and emergency cases, whatever their nature, and even allowing for the many difficulties at accident-and-emergency level. The deficiencies in the public hospital system are most evident in the area of elective medicine and chronic disease. This is not surprising when we have such a disproportionately high admission of acute compared to elective admissions to our major teaching and regional hospitals.[14] (See Table 2 on page 33.)

I believe that private patients, at least outside the public hospitals, do not necessarily receive better treatment than public patients. They may be admitted more quickly, but they may also be subjected to many more investigations, including the more elaborate ones,

TABLE 2: Variations in public/private and acute/elective admissions to specified hospitals in Ireland

	In-patients						Day Cases				
	ELECTIVE			EMERGENCY			TOTALS			TOTALS	
HIPE DATA 2004	Public	Private	Private as % of total	Public	Private	Private as % of total	Public	Private	Private as % of total	Total cases	Private as % of total	Private Beds
Dublin												
Tallaght	2,617	1,969	43%	10,264	5,019	33%	13,901	6,712	33%	40,482	34%	18%
Beaumont	3,761	2,287	38%	94,130	3,634	28%	24,411	5,169	17%	48,675	23%	17%
St James's	4,675	1,787	28%	12,416	3,290	21%	32,518	48	0%	54,734	9%	15%
St Vincent's*	3,574	481	12%	7,858	2,447	24%	16,238	261	2%	30,859	10%	9%
The Mater*	4,304	1,237	22%	6,635	1,988	23%	23,421	3,107	12%	40,692	16%	8%
Regional												
UCH Galway	6,837	3,399	33%	11,651	3,559	23%	12,722	4,444	26%	42,612	20%	18%
CUH	4,318	2,866	40%	10,911	3,272	23%	2,755	10,383	33%	52,505	15%	8%
MWRH, Limerick	2,701	2,545	49%	9,812	6,432	40%	10,783	7,448	41%	-39,721	41%	32%
Waterford	3,982	2,213	36%	14,578	5,033	26%	9,770	5,652	37%	41,228	24%	13%
Tullamore	1,732	783	31%	7,297	1,434	16%	6,573	2,766	30%	20,585	24%	12%
Drogheda	3,609	1,359	27%	11,913	4,456	27%	12,396	2,597	17%	36,330	23%	34%
Small												
Nenagh	249	134	35%	3,180	688	18%	1,541	1,145	43%	6,937	28%	32%
St John's Limerick	581	896	61%	1,368	894	40%	2,424	1,714	41%	7,877	44%	44%
Portiuncula	1,763	1,106	39%	5,512	2,255	29%	3,711	2,047	36%	16,394	27%	20%
Specialist												
Rotunda	4,370	2,949	40%	3,868	1,215	24%	880	1,014	54%	14,296	36%	29%
Holles St	4,476	4,390	50%	4,507	2,087	32%	820	170	17%	16,450	40%	36%
Coombe	4,691	3,694	44%	5,941	2,811	32%	864	1,114	56%	19,115	40%	32%
Crumlin	2,668	1,565	37%	4,640	1,939	29%	6,025	4,491	43%	21,328	37%	24%
St Luke's	1,178	436	27%	243	77	24%	2,489	1,524	38%	5,947	34%	20%
Croom, Limerick	856	830	49%	0	0	0%	598	1,351	69%	3,635	60%	35%

*Private hospital on site.

and to more intensive and prolonged treatment, than public patients – a situation which is consistent with the necessity for private hospitals to adequately use the expensive diagnostic facilities which they provide. The contention that private patients are subjected to over-diagnosis and over-treatment is supported by Ms Wren's evidence that private patients, at least within the public hospitals, are three times more likely to have a coronary angiogram than public patients. This is unlikely to be true in the acute coronary situation but may be so in elective cases. Whether this points to under-investigation of public patients or over-investigation of private patients is a moot point. I would consider the latter to be more likely.

In addition to the cost, private patients are subjected to other drawbacks because of excessive investigations. These include a risk of complications and of providing equivocal or false-negative or positive results which may conflict with sound clinical judgement. The private patient is not necessarily the privileged patient, as is generally believed. The international literature supports the view that private patients are subjected to a larger number of investigations than public patients, and may be over-managed.

Certainly any pretensions towards achieving a more equitable and more efficient health service may require government to move from a low-tax to a medium- or high-tax economy. There will be a continued increase in the proportion of GDP required for health. A new sense of social justice and idealism on the part of society, and effective accountability and audit on the part of the profession, as well as increased funding, will be required if we are to achieve a more just and equitable system which satisfies all.

As regards the health-care system in Ireland, we are currently in the melting pot, with the government's commitment to privatisation, the emergence of with-profit hospitals, and the marked trend towards the American system of health care, with its increasing cost, its inequities, its indifferent success in terms of life expectancy, and the serious threat to ethical practice among hospital owners, doctors and administrators.

In the absence of a one-tier system, the next-best solution would be private hospitals situated on the campus of public hospitals and staffed by the same medical personnel as the adjacent public hospital. The precedent for this arrangement is set by the St Vincent's Healthcare Group. Whatever system is adopted, it is imperative that the private, with-profit hospital should be rejected, not only to avoid the unacceptable conflict of interest between personal profit and patient care, but also to ensure that the care of the sick is the sole purpose of hospital services. Gaining profit from the treatment of the sick is inconsistent with the traditions of health professionals; indeed, the very concept of health insurance is solely aimed at providing us with the resources to ensure that we can always rely on society to support us when we are unwell. The president of the Royal College of Surgeons, Professor Niall

O'Higgins, in his 2006 presidential address, quoted a Harvard University researcher who questioned the principle of investor-owned care because it introduced a new value system that severed the communal roots and Samaritan tradition of hospitals.

The Labour Party, the Greens and Sinn Féin favour a one-tier system as part of their election policies, and Fine Gael may move in the same direction. There appears to be no great thrust on the part of the main government party to alter the inequitable two-tier system encouraged by Mr McCreevy's huge fillip to investors in private hospitals, nor does the minority PD Party's Thatcherite bent towards the American model appear to cause Fianna Fáil any great concern. Yet Fianna Fáil in its electoral manifesto promises to introduce an equitable, high-quality, one-tier system if re-elected to government.

According to the political observers with whom I have spoken, there may not be a great interest among the public in a one-tier system which would provide equal services to all, and this may make it difficult for the opposition parties to promulgate their policies. It may also be the basis for Fianna Fáil's coyness in advocating a one-tier system. The average citizen may think that Mary Harney has the quick answer by bringing in the profit-driven developers and investors, while few are conscious of the long-term implications of giving precedence to profit rather than patient care. No doubt the current prosperity of many of our citizens may account for the reported indifference of the electorate to a one-tier system. Perhaps we should be thinking of a one-tier private system entirely market-funded by health insurance, where 'extra' private care could be available for those who are able and willing to pay higher premiums. The government could insure the poor and the underprivileged by paying the insurance premiums. This solution is little different from the IMA proposal and, with co-operation of the medical profession, might take its cue from the Kaiser Permanente system in the United States.

Assuming a satisfactory service to public patients in a one-tier, tax-supported system, it is unlikely that a significant proportion of the population would pay for private medicine, apart from contributing towards private accommodation. The experience of our

European partners about the existence and usage of private hospitals would be of interest. It is difficult to believe that the current two-tier system can continue and still provide a satisfactory service for the 50 percent of the population who do not have health insurance. There is a limited amount of money available for health care in every society, even the more wealthy countries. The channelling of a large portion of the money available to the private sector will inevitably leave the public sector underinvested.

2

Private Hospitals and Public Welfare

Tussing and Wren conclude in their report (p11):

> Privatisation, meaning the substitution of for-profit forms of organisations for public or not-for-profit forms, poses still greater dangers to fundamental values. While one should not oppose privatisation in principle, one should be aware of the potential it has to do harm.

And again (p29):

> We argue for an equitable, universal health care system, with care delivered according to need and funded according to ability to pay.

Dr Christina O'Malley, president of the Irish Medical Organisation (IMO), criticised the current proliferation of private hospitals because of their failure to provide the comprehensive service available in our public institutions.[15] She talks about the cherry-picking propensities of private hospitals. We need to ponder the proliferation of private hospitals in Ireland and the encouragement provided by some of our political leaders for such hospitals.

In the early 1980s, I visited one of the largest and most prestigious private hospitals in the United States. I was met by the senior cardiologist. I enquired about the proportion of patients in coronary care in his hospital who were prescribed a coronary angiogram. He reckoned that about 90 percent of the patients had angiograms before they were discharged. In my own service in Dublin, not more than 10 to 15 percent had angiograms, and they were the minority who were deemed to be possible candidates for coronary surgery. I wondered why so many of his patients had the procedure performed. His reply was simple but unexpected. He said: 'Doc, I reckon that if I did not use the angio lab, my services would no longer be required by the hospital.'

This incident was my first reminder that there are more considerations in the medical world than simply patient care. Later in the 1990s, during a subsequent visit to New York, I read an exposé in the *Wall Street Journal* by a physician and administrator in the country-wide Columbia/HCA group of private hospitals.[16] He alleged that serious corrupt practices had been the norm in various hospitals in which he had previously been employed. The charges were being investigated by the federal authorities. These were private, with-profit hospitals, and there were 343 hospitals in the entire group at the time of the report. This group of hospitals subsequently changed its structure and management, and some of the hospitals were taken over by Triad Hospitals, which, with Johns Hopkins Hospital in Baltimore, are associated with the Beacon Clinic and Hospital, recently established in Sandyford in Dublin.

The Tenet group of hospitals has been subjected to massive fines because of serious and corrupt practices in its hospital at Reddin in California.[17] The fines include $500 million for unnecessary heart surgery, $1.5 billion for defrauding Medicare, and almost $400 million in settlements with individual patients. There are also reports from Australia that with-profit hospitals prescribe substantially more tests than are prescribed in the public hospitals,[18] a trend which is confirmed by Maev-Ann Wren in her 2003 report and repeated in her later publication with Dale Tussing in 2005.

It seems that the ethos of a with-profit hospital is inconsistent with the traditions of medical practice and of our profession. The possible abuse involved in over-diagnosis, over-treatment and unnecessary medicalisation of patients must be a contributory factor to the soaring costs of medical care in the United States, where the fact that the health-care system is the most expensive in the world is not reflected in the nation's health. The latest data from the United Nations states that the proportion of GDP spent on health in the US is 15.5 percent, while in Ireland it is just short of 9 percent, even after the massive increases in expenditure here during the last five years. As regards health-care costs in the future, Gerry Burke of the Bon Secours Hospital in Galway says that they will skyrocket because of increasing dependence on private facilities.[19]

I first published a note on the subject of with-profit hospitals in the *Irish Medical News* in August 2005. At about this time, there was a flurry of comment in the *Irish Times* on the subject from doctors and media commentators, who were mostly critical of Ms Harney's support for private medicine, and who placed particular emphasis on the adverse effect with-profit hospitals were likely to have on future services and on the ethical standards of our profession. One wonders what advice Ms Harney received and from whom she received it when she conceived the idea of creating eleven with-profit hospitals on the sites of our larger teaching and regional hospitals. Her proposal is certainly inconsistent with the recommendations of the many commission reports which were published about health during the last five years, and her judgement on the issue has raised considerable criticism among well-informed members of the profession and the public.

However, it is remarkable how little interest the medical profession at large has shown in the Harney initiative, nor do I have any information on Irish doctors' attitudes to privatisation. Sixty percent of doctors consulted in the UK are opposed to privatisation of the NHS, and there was immediate and trenchant medical and trade-union opposition to the UK government's advertising for applicants to provide private hospitals to supplement the NHS services. It was feared that this step would lead to the introduction of American-style hospitals run by American companies. The reaction by the public led to an immediate retraction by the Health Ministry.[20]

On the question of with-profit hospitals and the possible question of conflict of interest, I have been surprised at the relative lack of concern about with-profit hospitals shown by some of the consultant colleagues with whom I have spoken. The very concept of personal profit is inconsistent with the tradition of caring for the sick, but having doctors who are shareholders in profit-making hospitals points to a serious conflict of interest and must be unacceptable to the profession and disturbing to the public.

The only professional medical organisation to express its disquiet about with-profit private hospitals is the Adelaide Hospital Society. To the credit of this society, its director, Dr O'Ferrall, has published several well-informed articles in the medical and public press on the serious consequences of with-profit privatisation. Madeleine Spiers, president of the Irish Nurses' Organisation, writing in the *INO Journal*, has been critical of privatisation, and Dr Christina O'Malley, president of the IMO, has been particularly vocal in stating her concerns. Whether the views of the leaders of the INO and the IMO reflect the views of the membership is not clear. The silence of the IHCA on this issue may be based on its role in protecting the interests of its members, and I am not aware that the organisations representing GPs have entered the arena.

A meeting organised by the National Hospitals Action Group (originally set up to oppose the implementation of the Hanly report), and supported by the Adelaide Hospital Society, was held in Dublin on 26 November 2005. However, the meeting was poorly supported and there were few consultants present. Several speakers expressed their concern about the gradual Americanisation of our hospital services. On the same day, I received a pre-publication copy of ICTU's report on the Irish health system, which was researched and written by A. Dale Tussing and Maev-Ann Wren and was later published in book form. It is highly critical of privatisation.

I was compelled to write to the presidents of the two Royal Colleges because of the silence of their institutions on this and other health issues. At the end of November, I addressed a fellows' meeting of the Royal College of Physicians of Ireland on the subject of with-profit private hospitals, and I alluded to six reasons why I thought such hospitals would have an adverse long-term effect on our health service and on the ethos of our profession. These were an increase in cost to the public, a rise in insurance premiums, ethical problems, the collateral neglect of the public system, social divisiveness, and the cherry-picking advantages of the with-profit hospitals. The chairman of the College meeting was unable to discuss the matter in detail because the meeting was running late, but the response from the few who spoke was hardly positive.

One former president thought that it was not a matter for the College (although the College represents the great majority of physicians, north and south). On subsequently reading the seventeenth-century charter of the College, I found no mention of any matter except the qualifications necessary to become a Fellow, but penalties were prescribed for malpractice of various kinds and for conflict of interest, such as benefiting by being an apothecary or a vendor of medicaments or oils.

The late Dr David Mitchell, in his history of the College,[21] had this to say:

> In the meantime, the Royal College of Physicians of Ireland will continue to maintain and extend its influence for good medicine among its Fellows and Members. It should even aim to influence, in an unpartisan advisory role, the Minister for Health and her or his officers, and of course the media, which, all powerful, influence the public, among whom are doctors as well as patients, both present and future. This College can be exerted in many ways: from ex-officio appointments of Fellows to national or foreign health advisory bodies, to consultation with all formal or informal meetings of kindred bodies overseas.

He goes on to give the example of the College's success in its consultations with the minister on the subject of providing health notices on cigarette packages.

One member present at the meeting expressed his disapproval of doctors investing in with-profit hospitals. In private conversation after the meeting, a few colleagues were distinctly lukewarm about my views. Given the current decline in ethics, I expect they thought I was being quixotic. Only one colleague told me privately that he fully approved of my views. He was a full-time health employee of the North of Ireland's health service! It is surely depressing to think that our noble profession is selling its soul to mammon, and it is little consolation to know that we are simply following the trend among all elements of society. However, the president of the College undertook to raise the matter again at a further Council meeting, which he did at the next meeting of the Fellows in early March. Here he announced his intention to meet with the president of the Royal College of Surgeons and other representatives of the profession, presumably to discuss with-profit hospitals and other matters arising out of proposed changes in the health service.

There was a positive response from the president of the Royal College of Surgeons, who expressed serious concern about the way the profession was going when I wrote to him and when, later, we had an informal discussion about the subject. Although he was aware that some of his surgical colleagues may support Ms Harney's policies, he undertook to speak at a further meeting on the subject. Later, in his annual presidential address in February 2006, he spoke about the role of his College and of the profession in influencing the proposed changes in the health service. He expressed serious doubts about the concept of with-profit hospitals and announced his intention to consult with the president of the Royal College of Physicians and representatives of other organisations about the proposal by the current administration to encourage the private hospital sector. However, privatisation may soon reach a point of no return so that we shall find ourselves saddled with an American-style health service.

The councils of the two Colleges subsequently met. So far they have dealt mainly with teaching, training and professional standards. They have invited other groups involved with medical education to come together to define professional standards and to keep the health authorities informed on the need to maintain the highest level of professional training. I assume that any discussion about standards includes our ethical obligations, but I do not think that the question of with-profit hospitals has arisen in the course of discussion so far, nor has there been any overt criticism of the investors' profit motives introduced by Minister Harney.

It is surely wrong that a government can undertake such a major initiative affecting the health and well-being of Irish society without issuing a white paper on the subject and without consulting other political parties, the medical professions and other public interests.

It is astonishing how little interest individual doctors and nurses, and the political and academic medical institutions, have taken in current health-service proposals which, if implemented, will have a profound effect on future health care and on the ethics of medical practice. Equally, in the public and political domains, few seem concerned that our long tradition based exclusively on patient care will be seriously threatened by the pernicious drive for financial gain which is symptomatic of society today. I fear also that the lack of comment by the profession may be related to a vested interest in private practice, where the financial rewards are high, particularly in the high-tech field.

According to the recent Goodbody publication,[22] there were twenty-one private hospitals in the Republic in early 2005, with nine more under development and at least another six on the drawing board. It was estimated that 25 percent of the private hospitals existing in early 2005 were with-profit hospitals. More independent hospitals have been planned since then, and Ms Harney's intention to build eleven with-profit hospitals on the site of public hospitals seems to be evoking enthusiasm among potential investors The Mater Private Hospital has become a with-profit hospital, and both it and the Beacon have offered to build some of Ms Harney's proposed on-site private hospitals. Added to this is the announcement that Mount Carmel Hospital has recently been sold to a with-profit group.

With the continued depletion of the religious orders, it is highly likely that the group of four Bon Secours hospitals will be left to lay management, although there are members of the Order still on the board. I am informed by the current CEO, Pat Lyons, that the Bon Secours Order has sought agreement from the new board of management that the four hospitals must remain as non-profit hospitals, as heretofore. All profits will be retained and re-invested in the hospitals. The same condition will be applied to any new acquisitions by the group, which has been shortlisted for some of Ms Harney's co-location hospitals. Will the Bon Secours and the St Vincent's groups remain as the only hospitals in the country where the profit motive for personal and institutional investors will not prevail?[23]

There is also the problem of hospital chauvinism, where it is deemed necessary to provide special and expensive services which may not be justified because of the extent of the hospital's catchment area or the availability of similar facilities close by. We have the report of the intention to build a new private hospital in Adare which will provide a wide range of surgery, with six surgical theatres. Will it provide cardiac surgery? This hospital is planned to have a hundred beds. Will it have the necessary turnover of patients to justify advanced surgery? It is well established that hospitals with a relatively small turnover of heart-surgery patients have poorer results than those with large numbers of patients, and this must apply to many other surgical procedures. Will the Adare hospital attract enough well-trained staff? And will it be a with-profit hospital? If so, can we be satisfied that it will be run according to the highest ethical standards, and will the owners agree to independent auditing? Will it have the staff to deal with urgent problems, including patients who have been discharged by the same hospital? We are aware of the case histories of patients who, having undergone surgery or medical treatment in private hospitals, require unexpected follow-up attention and find that they must attend a public hospital because of lack of staff in the private institution.

The new Adare hospital will be less than ten miles from the regional hospital. The latter has 450 beds and eighty day-care beds. A new ninety-five-bed Blackberry Park hospital is also planned within the city. St John's Hospital, a non-profit private hospital with a hundred beds and Barrington's Hospital, with about sixty private beds, are also close by in the city of Limerick. Mary Harney has recently announced that one of the proposed with-profit private hospitals on the campus of a major public hospital may be built in Limerick,[23] adding a further hospital to the five that either exist or are planned. Is this multiplicity of hospitals serving a relatively small population really consistent with a realistic and efficient health service at a national level? And how rational are the many other proposals for private hospitals, such as the Whitfield, the Beacon, the Hermitage and the Ballymascanlon Clinic, to name but a few of the at least twenty facilities which exist or are planned? Are these being planned, or going into construction, without reference to the Department of Health, the HSE or insurance providers? And yet, in advertising their services, many of the new private hospitals claim to provide 'high-quality health care', implying, perhaps, that we in our tertiary and regional public hospitals have not always provided such care.

There are several other private clinical services going ahead, including the proposed health park in County Offaly, Touchstone Ltd, and the provision of mobile diagnostic services. Are they also receiving generous tax breaks, and are they part of the national health system planned by the department and the HSE? If we wish to provide an optimum health service for the people of Ireland, and one which is cost efficient, can we continue to invest willy-nilly in expensive private hospitals and clinics which are not included in the national plan for health, which are not referred to the central authority, and which have not been approved by the health-insurance industry?

Added to the multiplicity of hospitals in some regions, we have the anomaly of large numbers of private fee-paying patients in our public hospitals and of large numbers of public patients in our private hospitals, or being sent for investigation and treatment to other jurisdictions. The data on the number of private fee-paying patients in twenty of our public hospitals in 2004 were published recently.[24] (See Table 2, page 33.) They include five Dublin teaching hospitals, some regional and smaller hospitals, and a few specialist hospitals. St Vincent's University Hospital had the lowest proportion, at 12 percent, of private elective patients, but it has a non-profit private hospital on site under the same board of management. Four hospitals had between 20 and 29 percent, seven had between 30 and 39 percent, and eight had between 40 and 49 percent of private patients. In one hospital, Holles Street, 50 percent of the elective patients were private. The figures for day cases were more uneven. There were no cases in St James's and St Vincent's, but the other figures varied from 12 percent to 69 percent, with half at more than 30 percent. With the National Treatment Purchase Fund (NTPF) in situ since 2002, it would be interesting to know the statistics for 2005 for all public and private hospitals. Perhaps if the tortuous and bizarre planning by the health authorities continues along these lines, we might finish with a one-tier system based on private compulsory health insurance!

If Mary Harney were to place non-profit private hospitals on the campus of all our large tertiary public hospitals, with both hospitals under the same board of management, and if she were to discourage the building of new, expensive and fully equipped private hospitals off-site, there would be some sense in such a plan. While we might retain the independent private hospitals which have been established, we would have a two-tier system which would be acceptable because we would be assured that the same qualified consultant staff would be available to both sectors and that the investor profit motive would not affect our commitment to patient care. The arrangement at St Vincent's University Hospital is a good model.

Will the thirty-nine occupants of the Hermitage suites, or the consultants on the staff of the Beacon, have an association with a teaching or regional hospital? If Ms Harney could finance the private hospitals on site from central funds or by issuing fixed interest bonds to the public, she would overcome the main objection her 'misunderstood' critics have to her with-profit hospitals. And under these proposed circumstances, what would happen to the proliferation of independent with-profit hospitals and clinics which will be scattered around the country and which will eventually come home to roost with the taxpayers? Bearing in mind that Jimmy Sheehan's Hermitage hospital, with a hundred beds, is estimated to cost €110 million,[25] the eleven hospitals and the thousand private beds that Ms Harney envisages to reduce the numbers of private patients in the public sector would cost €1.2 billion – hardly a prohibitive sum when we currently have a revenue income of €2 billion in excess of the estimated revenue income for 2005. The other €1 billion could be used to improve community facilities for the elderly, the lonely, and the chronic sick and disabled. In this way, we could make a badly needed contribution to the social services, supporting the most disadvantaged and neglected members of our society while reducing the pressure on our public hospital beds.

It is difficult to understand why our criticisms of current health planning should prompt Ms Harney's to say that her policies have been received 'with some wild and ideological rhetoric' by those 'who choose to misunderstand this policy'.[26] This was at the First National Irish Private Healthcare Conference, a widely advertised meeting on private hospitals in one of our leading hotels, which was attended by few doctors but by many eager bankers, financiers and potential investors. Future health planning is not helped by such loudly publicised meetings. We might gain in understanding and tolerance if there was more communication between the minister and her critics. She was critical of her opponents on the issue of privatisation, and particularly about her support for with-profit hospitals. Maureen Browne, in her article reporting the meeting, was exuberant in her praise of privatisation.[27] She recounted the proceedings to a consultant friend of hers, 'who was delighted that I had gone to the conference and who agreed that it was the start of a new era in our health services. He was all for it: there would be choice and competition, not only for patients but also for medical and nursing staff.'

I am a critic of Ms Harney but would become a supporter if I was satisfied that all health care in this country was properly planned and coordinated, with the aim of establishing an equitable one-tier private health care service, or a two-tier system which shared the same medical staff and management without the investors' profit motive and without a proliferation of private, independent hospitals.

It is also difficult to understand the policy of the authorities in the case of the dialysis service. The HSE has accepted that further badly needed dialysis services are best provided by contracting out to the private centres, at a cost of an estimated €70,000 per patient per year. The Beacon service will cost €68,000 per year per patient, compared to an annual cost in Germany of €28,000 per year.[28] The Cabinet is currently studying the means of providing the necessary finance. This initiative is described by one correspondent as a solution but not a strategy, meaning, I suppose, that it is not a realistic part of a central, coherent plan. The increasing reliance on with-profit dialysis hospitals and dedicated centres is the result of the neglect of such services in the public sector and is further evidence of a dysfunctional approach to our national health problems. Is it the intention that, when the public dialysis service is developed sufficiently to be able to deal with all public patients, we will no longer require the facilities in the private sector? Or are we permanently locked in to this expensive solution to the problem?

Our health authorities today are adopting the health model current in the United States. A number of American companies have already arrived in Ireland, or are about to arrive here. Some of these hospitals may have doctors on the staff who are shareholders, a situation which should not be tolerated because of the obvious conflict of interest. The doctors in the private hospitals here may not be shareholders but may still find themselves under pressure, consciously or not, to maximise the use of elaborate and expensive investigations on which the with-profit hospital depends for survival.

In 2005, after publication of the Goodbody report, Ms Harney announced her plan to build eleven with-profit hospitals on the sites of public hospitals in various parts of the country, and it was announced in the media that the first two such hospitals were in the planning stage, probably in Limerick and Waterford.[29] Further, a report in *Medicine Weekly*[30] stated:

> Tánaiste Mary Harney's controversial plan for the construction of new private hospitals on existing public hospital lands took a step closer with the recent issuing of tender notices for the construction of eleven such facilities.

The list of eleven sites is added, and this information is followed by:

> This list of hospitals is an indicative list and additional sites identified will be the subject of a separate tendering process.

Soon the proportion of with-profit hospitals will greatly exceed 25 percent, and some of our current non-profit private hospitals will become with-profit institutions as their religious owners sell out to private investors. We shall soon be left with few non-profit hospitals and with an unethical two-tier system, unless we substitute a different method of funding the private hospitals. These hospitals could be funded from central sources or by issuing fixed interest bonds offered to the public or to the financial institutions, thus eliminating any conflict of interest. What will happen to the many independent private hospitals which are already in the system or which are currently planned when Minister Harney's policy has been implemented?

The prospect of with-profit private hospitals provoked me to write to An Taoiseach Mr Ahern expressing my views on the subject. I stated my preference for a one-tier system of health care based on compulsory health insurance as the best solution to hospital problems but allowed that the two-tier system, without with-profit hospitals, would be acceptable if it was based on the model of the St Vincent's Hospital Group. Here three hospitals, including a large non-profit private hospital, are under the same board of management, with common medical staff and with the opportunity to share treatment and diagnostic facilities. Whilst the governance is different for St Colmcille, Leopardstown, and the Royal Hospital in the same area, these institutions work in close association with the St Vincent's Group and share some common medical staff. The grouping of hospitals country-wide in this manner, with a common board of management, would lead to more rational local services, to greater efficiency, and perhaps to achieving by evolution rather than revolution some of the more desirable objectives recommended in the Hanly report. Twelve possible hospital groups are feasible, each of which could have a common board of management:

- § Drogheda, Cavan, Dundalk, Monaghan, Navan
- § Letterkenny, Sligo
- § Galway, Ballinasloe, Castlebar, Roscommon
- § Mullingar, Tullamore, Portlaoise
- § Limerick, Ennis, Nenagh
- § Cork public hospitals, Bantry, Mallow, Tralee
- § Waterford, Cashel, Clonmel, Kilkenny, Wexford

§ St Vincent's, St Michael's, Loughlinstown, St Vincent's Private, Leopardstown
§ Tallaght, Naas
§ St James's
§ Mater, Connolly
§ Beaumont

Children, maternity and other specialist hospitals might be governed along similar lines or might be associated with the larger groups.

Ms Harney's NTPF initiative, and her proposal to encourage the building of with-profit hospitals, encompass policies which may be expedient in solving some of our current problems but which lack foresight about the long-term implications of these policies in the context of cost, the perpetuation of an iniquitous health care system, and a decline in the ethical standards of health professionals. Instead of adopting a single-tier compulsory insurance system, we will be encumbered by the worst aspects of the American system. The disastrous policies now being promulgated by Ms Harney could not succeed without the indolence and lack of vigilance of the medical organisations and institutions. It is a question of bad legislation by politicians backed up by civil servants who act with little insight into affairs of health, and less into the adverse effect a deterioration in professional ethics will have on patient care and on cost; those who have – or should have – such insights remain silent and not consulted. And on the subject of cost, a future government, in introducing a one-tier system, may be faced with the same massive compensation to buy out the investors in the government and independent private hospitals as is the current government in buying out the investors in the National Toll Roads Company.

I have written twice to the Medical Council during the last three years enquiring about its attitude to practising colleagues who may be shareholders in with-profit private hospitals. This is a matter which ought to be brought into the public arena as well as being discussed more openly within the profession. The Council's stated statutory function is, among others, to protect the public from medical incompetence and abuse. As a profession, we are rightly responsible for our own standards, and the best protection our patients have is the medical profession's jealous concern for its own reputation.

On each occasion I wrote to the Council, I was referred to its published ethical guidelines, but it seems that the Medical Council will not intervene, nor will the Council express an opinion about specific professional or ethical acts unless a direct complaint is received from a member of the profession or the public. However, there are circumstances where it would be invidious to name any individual or group. Fortunately, under the presidency of Dr John Hillery, the Council is now showing greater concern about the standards of medical practice and of the need to maintain the public's trust in the medical profession.

Thanks to Mr McCreevy, who in 2002, as Minister for Finance, introduced substantial tax breaks to investors in new with-profit hospitals, we are facing the rapid Americanisation of our health system, a system which is at variance with that of the North of Ireland and of other members of the European Union. Barry Desmond, writing of his experience in Europe, where he was eleven years as an MEP and on the European Board of Auditors, states that Ireland is the only member of the expanded Union which has an inequitable health system.[31] Has Mr McCreevy also granted tax privileges for the refurbishment of some of our established with-profit hospitals, such as the Blackrock Clinic and the Mater Private Hospital? Strangely, the Department of Finance has rescinded such tax incentives in the future in all areas except in the case of private hospitals. Already, the taxpayer has lost huge sums to those investing in tax-incentive projects. Mr Cowen, the current Minister for Finance, must have yielded to the influence of the Minister for Health on this issue.

Then Minister for Finance Charlie McCreevy's measure, which is leading to the with-profit policy, came in response to lobbying by a doctor and a developer who had an interest in promulgating the private sector. Mr McCreevy's concession was passed by stealth. It was introduced not in the Budget but at the tail end of the parliamentary discussion on the Finance Act, without any prior notice to the members of the Dáil. Because of its method of introduction, its significance for future health legislation was not appreciated at the time by the TDs present, the medical profession and the public, but it has now come home to roost, with the proliferation of with-profit hospitals.

This political support for private hospitals was provided by Mary Harney when she introduced the NTPF in 2002 and when she proposed the building of ten (now eleven) with-profit hospitals on the sites of public hospitals. Mr McCreevy's response to lobbying by a few doctors reminds us that parliament may be losing out to lobbyists in relation to some aspects of legislation. It is a subversion of the principles of democracy and is an abuse which should be resisted by parliament. Senator Fergal Quinn has expressed such a view in an article in the *Irish Times*.[32]

We should have a single-tier health service in Ireland, along the lines of some of our European partners. It is the only system which is consistent with equity, and it may also be less costly than the two-tier system envisioned by Minister Harney. Ms Harney's proposals are even less acceptable than our old two-tier system, where the private sector was provided by religious or lay organisations and where patient care was the only consideration. We are currently proceeding along a rudderless course: hospitals are proliferating without any central planning or control by the government or the HSE, and despite the recommendations in the Hanley report, we are failing to reduce the numbers or the functions of some secondary-level hospitals. How can a wealthy person or group of investors decide to build an expensive hospital facility in the countryside without reference to government and without bringing chaos into our health-delivery system? Is departmental policy, presumably representing the policies of government, really based on a well-thought-out plan for the future?

The IMA working party report of 1974 was published in the Irish Medical Journal in 1975. It was a reasonable model for our hospital system as it existed at the time – a one-tier compulsory insurance scheme – but would require more research and a detailed examination of some of the European systems before being implemented. We have the precedent for such a successful service in some of the European countries, particularly the Scandinavian countries, and France and Switzerland. Under a single-tier service, private hospital facilities could be provided to those who wished to pay for extra comfort and privacy, but taxpayers' money should only be committed to the public sector. In some of the European countries with a one-tier system, there are at least some elements of private practice, including with-profit hospitals. Trends in these countries should be studied, as some appear be moving towards privatisation. A one-tier system would be compatible with the system in the North of Ireland, where co-operation is already taking place in the hospital services and where common research programmes relevant to both jurisdictions are being organised between our Health Research Board and its equivalent in the North.

It is unacceptable that our health minister, who may have little insight into the ethos of the caring professions, can threaten our age-long ethical traditions by introducing a system of with-profit private hospitals without a government white paper on the subject and without wider consultation with the public and the representatives of the medical professions. It is far too important an initiative to adopt without being aware of the serious consequences it may have on our public health services and on future taxpayers.

3

THE MEDICAL PROFESSION

There has been an appreciable decline in clinical medicine during my six decades in clinical practice. This has been particularly evident in the practice of cardiology, where the precise diagnosis of many cardiological conditions was based on the traditional use of eyes, ears and hands, and where reliable and confident prognostic and appropriate treatment decisions could be made with little more that an ECG – and even this test was not always necessary. This decline in the clinical tradition pertains in some other areas in medical practice too, and inevitably leads to a neglect of the disciplines of history-taking and physical examination, and in the training of young doctors in the fundamentals of diagnosis and the understanding of patients.

Huge advances have been made during the last sixty years in the diagnosis and treatment of some medical conditions, thanks to advances in technical methods, but the pendulum of diagnostic tests has swung too far, in that it is now becoming the custom to do unnecessarily complicated tests even on patients who require nothing more than a good clinical opinion. The very high proportion of normal tests which we see in our diagnostic centres can be attributed to the large number of patients who present with complaints which should be easily identified by a general practitioner trained in clinical medicine, and without any further enquiry than a careful history and a physical examination. Symptoms and signs generate far more powerful diagnostic information than we can ever hope to derive from the laboratory. Simple clinical data (such as the nature, location and distribution of pain; circumstances of onset of symptoms; precipitating factors; and the association with other symptoms) can define the investigations, which may be relevant and should provide the trained clinician with clear indications as to what tests are required to assist in diagnosis and in deciding prognosis and treatment. The close contact with the patient which is inherent in good clinical practice is essential in order to achieve accurate diagnosis and high standards of care, to ensure trust among patients, and to reduce litigation. It has been shown that doctors who spend more time talking to their patients in the clinical setting are less likely to be sued.[33] We have to face the reality that, thanks to the internet and to better education among the masses, patients will be better informed about medical matters and their own problems, and will only be satisfied by a high degree of professionalism.

The burgeoning cost of medical care is such that, given no financial limitation, we might eventually leave little for other public services. It is obvious that spending on health care will need to be limited, and that such limitations will affect clinical practice. With our fragmented system, and particularly with a profit-making private sector, there is little opportunity for slowing the current semi-exponential increase in health costs. Indeed, with current policies, the increase in costs may accelerate. Nor does it seem to matter that the benefits of medical intervention may be approaching the point where some interventions are no longer cost-effective. An example here is the increasing tendency to provide aggressive and invasive measures in treating the old, where the benefit may not be justified by the physical and psychological consequences of such intervention. Partial payment by all insured patients for medical services, combined with more active community provisions at GP level, would reduce our dependence on expensive hospital services.

Incentives to admit patients to hospital must be examined and controlled. We may have to follow the British in imposing strict budgetary constraints on hospitals, and doctors may need to be less interventionist in dealing with terminally ill patients. We also need to reverse the current trend away from clinical bedside medicine and to be stricter about following the tenets of evidence-based practice. These ideas may be quixotic and pie-in-the-sky, but clearly doctors need to reconcile their professional obligations with the hard facts of limited financial resources. Society needs to adopt the cultural and behavioural changes which may provide a more rational approach to the questions of health and illness. Perhaps a useful first step would be to change the term 'health service' to 'sickness service' and to describe government policies aimed at better health in the community – better exercise facilities, better nutrition, education aimed at physical and psychological health – as our health service!

It is not realised how profound an impact the increasing reliance on tests is likely to have on the cost of the health services in terms of staff, equipment, space and technical resources – even before mentioning the occasional risk to patients. The €200 million addition to St Vincent's University Hospital has a new A&E department but is otherwise designed to provide improved technical, administrative and outpatient facilities. There are no additional beds for elective patients and only short-term beds for acute admissions. These facilities may of course lead to better and easier opportunities to investigate patients at an outpatient level.

Many tests lack adequate sensitivity and specificity, thus providing false negatives and false positives. Not infrequently, the results of these tests may be equivocal, leading to further time being spent on the medical treadmill. When we add the effect of the expanding high-tech medicine to the growth in litigation, the ageing population, the significant role of iatrogenic, or doctor-induced, disease, the commercialisation of medicine, and Illich's prospect of a prolongation of death through modern medical intervention, we must have serious doubts about designing a health service which will satisfy both the public and the Exchequer.

The commercialisation of investigations can be noted in several areas. Apart from the pressure on doctors to employ more investigations by the medical industry, hospitals and clinics vie with each other to provide every available test which might be deemed to be essential in diagnosis. These may be necessary in a limited number of cases, but the natural history of this phenomenon is that, if the facility is there, it is a simple matter to avail of it in a routine rather than in an indicative manner, and thus to encourage the creation of a waiting list. Particularly worrying is the recent advent of the private, and sometimes mobile, diagnostic facility, such as magnetic resonance imaging (MRI), by commercial, profit-earning companies. Without independent audit, private medicine could lead to major problems in terms of cost, poor practice and unacceptable ethical problems. It should be illegal for such services to function in the health domain without strict and independent audit, and this should be provided by the forthcoming Health Information and Quality Authority (HIQA) of the HSE, regardless of whether the service is provided in the public or private sector, or the hospital or clinic is independent of the central health authority.

The commercial, profit-making MRI Centre reported in March 2006 a profit of €295,000 for 2004.[34] It has its registered office in Barrington's Hospital in Limerick and apparently owns MRI Centre – Galway Ltd. It is stated that there is one owner only. Whether the owner is a member of the medical profession is not stated. Is this service subject to independent audit? Should such private, with-profit medical treatment and diagnostic facilities be provided without independent surveillance of standards of practice by GPs or specialists? Should part of our insurance premiums go to private investors?

There are many examples of poor management arising from an excessive reliance on tests. There is a catch-22 situation evident in current medical practice – the increasing reliance on tests as the basis of diagnosis leads to an inevitable decline in clinical practice and impairs the doctor's insight into the patient's holistic problems. The usual justification put forward for the excessive use of tests is that it is necessary for medico-legal reasons. But this is sloppy thinking. If we talk to our patients and, where necessary, to the relatives, and if we are good clinicians, and if we only prescribe tests when they are perceived to be relevant to diagnosis, prognosis and treatment, it is highly unlikely that we will find ourselves in the law courts because of failure to do inappropriate tests. Added to this, effective audit, still awaited and badly needed, will reduce the risk of litigation in our hospitals.

It is also stated that patients demand tests; but a caring and competent doctor, through appropriate explanation and reassurance, can usually deal with such pressures. The growth of high-tech investigations, led by the mindset which gives precedence to tests rather than careful clinical analysis, is putting the cart before the horse. It is a major factor in the current exponential increase of health service cost and is a compelling reason for a return to clinical medicine as the basis of good practice. It is also a compelling reason for proper audit in our hospitals aimed at controlling the sloppy use of diagnostic and treatment facilities. Liam Murray, head radiographer at St John's Hospital in Limerick, believes that 40 percent of chest X-rays which are ordered are unnecessary and do not conform to good clinical practice.[35]

The excessive availability of complex investigations may also lead to poor and sometimes incompetent practices. I shall give one example illustrating this point. A well-known Irish professional golfer visiting the United States in 2005 heard about the new cardiac CT test (technically called a sixteen-channel cardiac computed tomography). This is an important advance in diagnostic radiology. It can identify blockages in the coronary arteries as efficiently as the invasive coronary angiogram and in some cases may have advantages over angiography. The golfer decided to have one during his stay. Apparently a stenosis was identified, and he was advised to have it treated by angioplasty and stenting. The X-ray and the subsequent procedure must have been expensive, and the angioplasty is not without some risk of complications. He was informed that, without the intervention, he was at risk of a heart attack.

Indeed, the use of this test may not be without its problems, as is confirmed by a recent paper in the *Journal of the American Medical Association*,[36] which shows that the test can lead to false-positive and false-negative results, and thus can lead only to clinical confusion. These findings are also reported by other researchers. A more advanced model of the CT scan has been installed at the Blackrock Clinic; this scan may be less liable to false-positive and false-negative results. Nonetheless, the more we advance the frontiers of high-tech medicine, the more likely it is that false-positive and false-negative findings may lead to further tests, and sometimes to confusion or inappropriate treatment.

None of the clinical trials available to us have confirmed that there is ever a need for invasive treatment of a coronary stenosis which is asymptomatic in an apparently clinically healthy person. Like all apparently healthy people, the person in such a case should be advised to avoid the well-known risk factors for coronary disease. By being sensible in matters of lifestyle, he would be highly unlikely to develop coronary heart disease; patients who have little to show in a cardiac scan but who smoke and have an abnormal lipid profile are much more likely to suffer a heart attack. An unstable coronary endothelium with little or no stenosis may be vulnerable to thrombosis in such high-risk cases. Despite the angioplasty, the golfer in question must not think that he can now afford to be complacent about his lifestyle.

Our golfer may have read the banner headlines in *Time* magazine in September 2005, where the correspondent describes how a casual cardiac scan led to an asymptomatic man having an angioplasty and stent, 'thereby preventing what could have been a heart attack'. The article adds: 'what that means is that millions of patients will probably get the treatment that better matches their condition'. In other words, after a routine cardiac CAT scan, they can be prescribed appropriate medical treatment or invasive procedures if they have an asymptomatic stenosis; and the millions who have normal scans can 'feel confident that they don't need statins and other medications, along with their potential side effects', presumably even if they smoke and have an abnormal blood cholesterol profile! Without a history of heart disease, no healthy person requires drug treatment for a high-cholesterol profile unless this profile fails to respond to healthy-eating habits and an appropriate aerobic-exercise programme. We are unlikely to develop coronary heart disease, and even more rarely require heart surgery or angioplasty, if we follow the simple rules of healthy living. All this simply confirms that, in achieving a healthy and long-living society, education is more important than an elaborate health service devoted to non-acute illness.

You may be sure that, in their efforts to prevent heart disease, the physicians and radiologists who advocate routine CT scans in healthy, asymptomatic people have little insight into the potential for preventive medicine through less expensive and more rational means. For the sake of their patients' welfare, they would be better occupied in counselling their patients about their lifestyles. If every middle-aged adult were advised to have such a prophylactic cardiac CT scan, the health services would be in complete chaos and would require 100 percent of our GDP. No matter how advanced we are in developing sophisticated diagnostic methods, we should not provide unnecessary medical or invasive treatment for patients who are free of symptoms and otherwise risk-free. Such abuses are at the basis of our current escalating health costs.

Medicine, like nursing, is primarily about helping people and, no matter how sophisticated and important are the many investigations which are part of medical practice nowadays, we cannot afford to distance ourselves from our patients. The dilemma which we face is how to maintain our clinical role and to be prudent and judicious in the use of tests. Hence the urgent need for audit. Our clinical competence and integrity would also be assured if tests were in general carried out by dedicated technicians or nurses and not by clinicians. The Kaiser Permanente system has proven how we can be much more conservative about investigations, to the benefit of patient care and of cost.

During my later years in hospital, as therapeutics and the choice and availability of investigations became more complex, much of the waste in prescribing and in arranging investigations could be attributed to lack of supervision of young non-consultant hospital doctors (NCHDs) in training – one argument against our current consultant contract. In my sixteen-bed coronary care unit and recovery ward, we had a rule that drugs (apart from mild painkillers and sedatives) and investigations could not be ordered without the approval of the registrar or myself, unless prescribing was directed by a printed protocol. It is my belief that the profession has failed to keep abreast of drug technology. The overuse of drugs and, to a lesser extent, the inappropriate use of drugs is evident in current everyday practice. In the late 1980s, my resident staff and I published a paper which confirmed that one hundred successive patients discharged from the cardiac department in the hospital were on fewer drugs than they had been at the time of their admission.[37] Our experience confirmed that many patients admitted to coronary care were already on long-standing medical treatment and that a minority of the population make up the majority of hospital patients.

The inappropriate use of drugs raises complex issues, but these issues are beyond our control unless we have proper audit and accountability. Current obligatory postgraduate training programmes may be justified and may help to maintain the standards of practice but, without proper audit and accountability, it is unlikely that we will be able to reach high standards of prescribing investigations and treatment. Much of the overuse of drugs can be attributed to the pervasive pressure of the drug industry, ably abetted by the medical journals and newspapers.

Another contributory factor to the decline in clinical medicine is our method of choosing applicants for entry to the medical profession. The points system is advantageous because it greatly simplifies the choice of candidates and therefore suits the medical faculties in our universities. It also ensures that there is gender and social equality in the process, and therefore satisfies the liberal wing and the politically correct. But it has serious disadvantages in that the academic achievements of candidates bear little if any relationship to their suitability for a career in a caring profession such as medicine. A more important factor in selecting candidates for medical training is the applicant's motive in seeking a career in medicine. Those who are interested in becoming part of a caring profession because they have a genuine interest or tradition in the welfare of others are much less likely to become drop-outs during or after their training period, and are better qualified to function in the hands-on clinical setting. By virtue of including appropriate social, psychological, academic and personality factors in assessment, we are likely to find candidates who are more committed to a medical career. While the proper assessment of candidates may require substantially more time and input by the medical faculties, this can be done by using appropriate questionnaires and interviews, and would benefit the professional standards of doctors and the welfare of patients.

There is also a need to consider the wider education of students if we in the medical professions hope to retain our traditional counselling and caring role. The gradual decline of the humanities in secondary and tertiary education, including ethics in its wider and practical sense, must have a deleterious effect on our profession in the future. No doubt in our materialistic and secular society, any reference to the humanities will be considered irrelevant.

In the early 1970s, medical students' close contact with patients at the clinic and the bedside, which was an integral part of undergraduate training, began to wane, and to be replaced by the tutorial and the classroom. In my daily work at the hospital, I had always been attended by students, whether on ward rounds, on consultations or in the outpatient service. By 1988, when I retired, I seldom saw a medical student, apart from at the one lecture on cardiology I was scheduled to give every fortnight – although by then I had been appointed to a Chair by the university. While the practice of medicine thirty or forty years ago was clearly less complex, with a greater emphasis on the clinical approach, the students in these earlier years were closer to the patients, having spent six months in residence and having attended ward rounds and outpatient clinics as part of their education. They were more mature and more clinically adept than their modern counterparts. Compared to the typical recently qualified doctor in my early years, the young pre-registration doctor who joins the hospital staff after graduation is nowadays just starting out on the learning curve of clinical medicine and patient management. Forty years ago, we spent all our working hours with patients. Many consultants still do, but medical students certainly do not.

In Ireland, we have the added problem of our consultants' contract, which has been criticised as too generous by Maev-Ann Wren and other critics, and there is little enthusiasm among our consultants about audit, particularly in the private sector. We do hear talk of our centres of excellence, but how can we confirm that they are centres of excellence if we are not provided with information about their standards and results?

Doctors insist on clinical freedom but there is too much waste in the use of drugs, too much access to routine tests, too much variation in diagnostic and therapeutic practice, and too much freedom among doctors in training to order drugs and investigations without proper supervision from their seniors. Clinical freedom may have been appropriate in the past, when the number of drugs was limited to relatively harmless and inexpensive stimulants, potions and nostrums, and when diagnostic and therapeutic decisions involved little expense and less harm to patients, but today, with ever-expanding drug technology and a dramatic increase in the number and cost of diagnostic procedures, the days of clinical freedom, of doctors practising without accountability, must surely be over. In our efforts to cure or to restore health, we doctors would, if we had our way, be oblivious to the practical limits of health expenditure, while greater benefits in terms of health and life expectancy could be achieved at a fraction of the cost by public-health education and appropriate social engineering. The current wide divide in the health and mortality experience of the different social classes is largely the consequence of different levels of education, and not of deficiencies in the health service.

Herein, however, lies our dilemma. We must continue to look after the sick with the greatest possible commitment and professional skills. If we hope to do so within the practical limits of our health services, we must divest ourselves of the concept of clinical freedom, at least at the personal level, and must be seen to conform to the highest standards of practice. We must learn to balance benefit in medical terms with financial cost and the cost of possible physical and psychological side effects – not an easy task in the clinical setting. However, cost control is now part of the British health system, through the imposition of strict budgeting on hospitals and community practice, and the cost of health services is preoccupying economists and politicians in many other Western countries, including the United States. The trend towards providing with-profit private hospitals may seem a facile solution to some of our cost problems, but such a solution will have exactly the opposite effect, quite apart from its damaging influence on the Samaritan tradition of our profession.

While the prospect of audit is greeted with mixed feelings by consultants because it may impair their concept of clinical freedom, peer review and audit in our hospitals can maintain clinical freedom at a corporate level. Because we are responsible for our patients' lives and well-being, and because we are capable of doing serious harm as well as good, we must be accountable for our actions.

There are compelling reasons for more audit and accountability by doctors in the private institutions, including private investor–led companies providing diagnostic services directly to doctors in private hospitals and general practice. At least in the larger public teaching hospitals, consultants, resident staff and other health professionals may work closely together. Conferences are held to discuss surgical and medical cases which require careful diagnostic and therapeutic analysis. Without these circumstances and proper audit, no institution can claim to be a centre of excellence. Because of possible added pressure by owners on the consultant in the private hospital, practice assessment should be mandatory. In the context of the increasing cost and complexity of medical practice, it is unlikely that we can achieve much-needed improvements in our health services without effective audit of all aspects of the system. The provision of proper audit can best be provided by the medical profession itself, but this will require changes in doctors' current attitude towards accountability.

Consultants with a contract of ten sessions a week should have the necessary time and facilities to maintain an audit system. I find a somewhat negative attitude to audit among some colleagues. It creates too many administrative problems and is time-consuming; in practice, it may receive little more than lip service. By contrast, in our maternity hospitals, audit was and is a fundamental part of the service. In these hospitals, results were reported annually at a meeting which was open to the profession and the public, and which was convened at the Royal Irish Academy of Medicine. It is certain that we owe the worldwide reputation Ireland acquired in reproductive medicine and the high standards of the obstetric service to the mastership system, which has been in existence without change for 250 years, and to the comprehensive annual reports published by our obstetricians.

Dr John Hillery, president of the Medical Council, writing in the *Irish Times* on 28/2/06, stresses the necessity of effective audit and peer review of medical practice in the current circumstances, where doctors can do so much harm to their patients and their pockets, to the taxpayers, and to the reputation of the medical profession. He describes a system of random choice of practitioners who would be asked to volunteer (at least for the present) to have their standards of practice examined by a chosen group of experts. It is likely that his proposal is intended more for GPs. Dr Hillery's intentions are excellent, but in practice they might be difficult to implement, and might be best replaced by in-house audit within the GP co-ops, or by a system of drug-usage inspection, as was recommended by the Cohen Committee in the British NHS.

The audit of consultants might be organised along different lines. A properly constituted hierarchical system of governance should exist in every large hospital, where a chief of staff and a small executive would have responsibility for audit. Added to this, we should have appropriate access to the Hospital In-patient Enquiry (HIPE) system, first established by the Medico-Social Research Board in 1969 but subsequently moved to the ESRI after the MSRB was subsumed by the newly established Health Research Board in 1986. HIPE measures of treatment and of outcomes are limited. It is strictly a health-information system and may need additional input in order to act as an effective audit method; nonetheless, it is sufficient to provide clues or raise suspicions about inappropriate practice. Currently, HIPE does not include the private hospitals. It is essential that all hospitals should by included, and that the scheme be made compulsory. While the strictest confidentiality needs to be maintained, it should be possible to detect any aberrant practice, whether at an institutional or individual level. Clearly the newly constituted Interim Health Information and Quality Authority (IHIQA) may fill an important role in audit and in maintaining confidentiality. Hopefully, its authority will extend to all aspects of the health service, including private hospitals which have been established independent of the central health authority and without consultation with the insurance industry.

Derek Lambert, in a letter to the *Irish Times* published on 3/3/06, at the time of the Neary inquiry, suggested that, if the HIPE system of surveillance had been in full and effective operation in Ireland at the time, the fact that the doctor at the centre of the inquiry had carried out excessive numbers of post-pregnancy hysterectomies would have been obvious. Lambert might also have added that such a system might have relieved many well-meaning but invariably victimised whistle-blowers of their unenviable task. Because of the inhibitions inherent in reporting on colleagues, it is understandable why so many of Dr Neary's peers, and those on the staff of the Drogheda Hospital, failed to report his aberrant practices. According to a Supreme Court decision, there is no legal protection for clinical audit material in Ireland – a further source of concern to the potential whistle-blower.[38]

It was announced recently that Mary Harney proposes to set up a hospital inspectorate to examine competence assurance as part of the new Medical Practitioners Bill.[39] According to Judge Maureen Harding Clark, in her report on the Neary case, mentioned in the same article, there might also be a need for competence assurance for other, non-medical hospital staff. If audit becomes too complex in its planning, it may be self-defeating. I believe that, with proper consultant structures and internal audit, added to the universal use of HIPE, the inspectorate could function simply as the body responsible for the surveillance of HIPE. Perhaps it is proposed that the IHIQA should take on this role.

There is another benefit to be gained from effective internal audit in our hospitals, where a proper consultant structure is in place, and by the comprehensive working of the HIPE programme. Both forms of surveillance would substantially reduce the volume and cost of medical litigation in the community. It would also help to reduce the incidence of iatrogenic disease. The savings from a reduction in litigation should at least cover the costs of the HIPE system.

The profession needs to face up to the realities of the common contract, which we can hardly expect to continue in its present form. Tussing and Wren, in their report, describe the consultants' contract as deeply flawed, and believe that it is one of the causes of our dysfunctional service. They say:

> Consultants are paid public salaries while treating private patients. They are not accountable administratively or clinically. (p14)

Consultants' extraordinary degree of autonomy and excessive delegation to NCHDs raise serious management problems and have been criticised in a series of studies. (p20)

The number of consultants who take significant advantage of the access to the NCHDs must be small and confined to a few of our larger hospitals. The right of consultants to delegate a significant part of routine public work to the doctors in training, especially in case of emergencies, should no longer be continued, but changes in rostering and availability are some aspects of practice which need consideration. Consultants who practise in private hospitals off-site should not expect the same income for their more limited commitment to the pubic service, nor should consultants who earn a large income from private patients within the public hospital expect no limitation of their public salary. Where possible, and particularly in the large public hospitals with private hospitals attached, consultants should be confined to the hospital campus. Also, the cost of clinical research should not be a charge on the public service, whatever about the cost of teaching.

According to Ms Wren, consultants can earn more than €500,000 annually. I would estimate that these are the relatively few who perform invasive investigations, who are directors of major laboratories, or possibly those in a few surgical specialities. A large income is not uncommon among those in other professions and in business, and is not any more unacceptable in our highly trained and skilled medical specialists. In Canada, consultants' fees are capped. While this is unlikely to appeal to consultants in Ireland, it would at least reduce the frenetic activity of some of our busier colleagues, who may have difficulty controlling private practice. It would leave them with more time and leisure to talk to patients and relatives, and to maintain audit.

The health service in Ireland and in other Western countries would surely benefit if many of the more specialised investigations were carried out by dedicated technicians. This would lead to more efficiency, would certainly be less costly, and would remove the possibility of conflict of interest. It would also reverse the current trend away from clinical practice among physicians who frequent the laboratory rather than the ward.

Table 2 (see page 33) records the proportion of private and public patients admitted to some of our public hospitals in 2004, including acute and elective admissions.[40] The number of elective private patients greatly exceeds the 20 percent allowed under the common contract. Although the NTPF commenced in 2002, it is probable – although by no means certain – that this high number of private elective admissions in the public sector may fall with the further implementation of the scheme. It is hard to envisage a realistic health service where such a large proportion of private patients occupy public beds and so many public patients occupy private beds as is currently the case under the NTPF. One might have expected a greater proportion of acute admissions of private patients, rather than elective patients, to the public sector. Might the consultants have an influence in admitting such large numbers of elective patients? And why are so many day-care private patients admitted to our public hospitals – almost certainly because of the absence of adequate private day-care investigative and treatment facilities for such patients. Perhaps the bed may be unnecessary in many such cases, although it may be required in order to satisfy optimum insurance coverage.

It would be important to analyse the reasons for such high private elective admissions to the public hospitals. Is it likely that they, like the emergency admissions, cannot be dealt with in a private hospital? How have we arrived at such a convoluted solution to our health-delivery problems? Why do we have a limit of 20 percent of private patients in public hospitals and yet virtually no notice is taken of such an arrangement, while public patients are on a waiting list from which the minister arranges that they are admitted to a private hospital – often the same hospital on whose admission list they have been waiting? The situation is bizarre; perhaps the only quick solution is to establish a one-tier private system for all, supported by health insurance, where the premiums of the less privileged are paid from central funds or supported by the issuing of government bonds.

With such a high number of private patients in our public hospitals, it would seem desirable to claim a proportion of the private fees for research, and for other professional and academic purposes for those health professionals attending the patients. This is the rule in some other countries.

It is unlikely that real order can be brought into the health services here without some radical changes within the medical profession, and these changes would need to come from within the profession itself. Doctors have traditionally received the support of the Irish people when they are involved in controversy with politicians or other critics. The sympathy of the people is probably a product of the dedication of the profession to charitable work in the past, but the charitable role of the doctor is now less evident, and it is likely that our profession will not retain the affection and sympathy of our patients and politicians in the future when we are struggling with our adversaries.

Consultants in some of our larger hospitals are not organised in a hierarchical way, and as a result there is less accountability than necessary, and insufficient audit or attention to cost control. Many years ago, I proposed to our newly appointed professors of medicine and surgery at St Vincent's Hospital that we adopt a hierarchical system along the lines of the Cogwheel Report published in the United Kingdom nearly forty years ago.[41] Each department would have a rotating chairperson who would be an ex-officio member of the medical committee. The chairman of the committee would be elected by the consultants and would be appointed chief of staff for a limited tenure, say of five to seven years, rather along the lines of the mastership system, which has survived for more than 250 years in our maternity hospitals. He or she would be required to work closely with the administration and would receive sessional payments for such services. He or she would be ex-officio a member of the board of management of the hospital, would have equal status with the CEO, and would be responsible to management for the standards maintained by all medical colleagues. Through the medical committee, the chairman would have executive powers to deal with medical-staff problems, including the provision of satisfactory office and secretarial facilities for colleagues and for a system of audit and professional accountability, and discipline. The

Neary problem would not have arisen if the Drogheda Hospital had had a proper consultant structure along these lines.

In his presidential address to the Royal College of Surgeons in 2005, Professor Niall O'Higgins was critical of the loss of influence of consultants in hospital administration. The profession itself must share at least part of the blame for this unfortunate situation. Without the profession's leadership, our health services cannot be satisfactorily solved, but our profession has in many ways and in many hospitals lost its leadership in management and in its concern for a service which should be primarily patient-driven. The members of the medical profession as a whole, as well as their academic and professional institutions, are surprisingly passive and complacent in accepting Ms Harney's radical attempts to change the Samaritan ethos of our profession to a mercenary one, and hospital doctors' vital role in policy and management is being subsumed by an overbearing administration. The perception of the public must nowadays be that doctors' primary preoccupation is to ensure that they defend their own privileges. Looking back to the time before my retirement in 1988, many of us, both clinical and technical staff, were closely involved in administration, particularly of our own departments, and many of us who were closely associated with the Irish Medical Association and other areas of medical politics showed considerable interest in advancing a better-organised and more coherent health service. One of the many benefits which professional involvement in hospital administration brings is a better balance between administrator and medical and nursing staff, thus averting an overbearing bureaucracy.

In the past, we had closer and more harmonious relations with the lay administrators, and there was closer cohesion between all those concerned with hospital policy and management. One factor which accounts for our profession's decline in managing our hospitals has been the loss of clinical departments in some of our hospitals. This step was taken since my departure from hospital practice and must certainly be related to the current high proportion of acute admissions. Formerly, clinical specialists were responsible for a defined number of beds in the hospital wards, where, apart from emergency cases, patients were deemed to require the attention of the specialist in charge. We had close contact with a dedicated nursing staff, many of whom remained in the same department for years and who were intimately aware of patients' needs. The authority in the wards was the joint responsibility of the ward sister and the senior consultant in the department. Patients admitted as emergencies were, if necessary, subsequently transferred to the appropriate specialist elsewhere in the hospital.

Specialists who find themselves with patients scattered in various parts of the hospital and without a clinical base are disadvantaged for several reasons. Among other things, this fragmentation has loosened the close ties between doctor and nurse and has deprived many of the consultants of administrative responsibility, and to some extent of the consultant's pride in the institution. It is more difficult to define which consultant is in charge of the patient, and who may be responsible to the admitting GP, and this has had a damaging effect on the ethos of the hospital – a factor which is important for good hospital standards but is not always appreciated by the laity.

An institution is only as good as its component parts. Nelson, Bataldan and their colleagues in the United States published nine papers under the general title of *Microsystems in Health Care*.[42] Their theme was the importance of the morale, efficiency, leadership, caring qualities and inclusiveness of each microcosm, each clinical department, and how much high-quality departments could add to the status of the hospital in the community. These nine papers have their fair share of jargon, but they are essential reading for those who are concerned about hospital management, and the morale and responsibility of clinical consultants in our large hospitals. When we had our own departments devoted to specialist medicine and surgery, we invariably took pride in our department and its staff. We were a potential microcosm of a proud and caring institution and were inevitably more involved in hospital administration and hospital policy. There was closer cohesion with the administrative staff and, all around, a more palpable ethos in the whole institution.

In 2004, 4,055 elective and 10,305 emergency patients were admitted to the wards of St Vincent's University Hospital. In the same year, 4,586 elective and 15,283 emergency patients were admitted to the hospital in Tallaght.[43] The situation is little different in our other teaching and regional hospitals. Clearly, there are difficulties in restoring the clinical units in our general hospitals, largely because of the rather chaotic A&E situation and the difficulty in admitting elective cases, but every effort should be made to restore dedicated departments, at least when the A&E situation has improved and when the consultant structure is organised in a hierarchical manner in our larger hospitals.

Maev-Ann Wren contends that the current hospital services are doctor-driven. This may well be correct but, without wishing to dominate health policy and without resisting desirable political decisions with regard to health, doctors should continue to influence decisions about community and hospital practice. The answer to the president of the Royal College of Surgeons, who bemoaned his colleagues' loss of influence in hospital administration, lies in the consultants establishing a proper hierarchal structure in their hospitals, where they must be seen to maintain the highest standards of hospital management. I believe that consultants have only themselves to blame if they lose their leadership role in hospital organisation. The beneficial and essential role of the consultants in hospital management is evident in some of our provincial hospitals, including Sligo, Kilkenny and Clonmel.

The best and most efficient hospitals will be staffed by consultants who share administration with other medical professionals and lay managers, who have a pride in their institution, who are conscientious, and who are committed to the traditions and ethical standards of their profession.

While this essay is being written (June 2006), meetings between the Department of Health, the HSE, the IMO and the IHCA regarding a new contract for consultants are about to be resumed following a five-month delay. These meeting are likely to be further prolonged. They may be contentious because consultants will be required to make changes which will affect their current status, and the unlimited access to private practice currently enjoyed by some consultants may be curtailed in the future. Certainly it is difficult to believe that the current contract can continue if the wider problems within the service are to be solved. It will require an unusual degree of firmness and determination on the part of the politicians to find agreement with the medical organisations on desirable changes in the current common contract. Any fair-minded person would agree that the contract is exceptionally liberal in some of its terms. Hopefully, reasonable concessions will be considered when the doctors and health authorities return to their discussions.

4

THE NURSING PROFESSION

The changing financial and academic status of nurses in recent years has added significantly to the financial and organisational problems of hospitals. The move from the hospital to the university campus during the years of nurse training has deprived the hospital of valuable nursing input and has partially deprived the nurse at a sensitive time in her or his career of the vocational stimulus which is essential in a caring profession and which is derived from direct, hands-on patient care. Equally important has been the adverse effect of the change on the ethos of our hospitals because of the loss of our on-site training schools, and the inevitable reduction of the strong links which existed in all teaching hospitals between the nursing staff and its alma mater.

In my time at St Vincent's Hospital, our nursing school, first established in 1892, was highly regarded both nationally and internationally, and was an integral part of the hospital's proud history. It vanished overnight five years ago, as did the founders and owners of the hospital, the Sisters of Charity. With them went some of the spirit and pride which were the source of our loyalty to a great institution. In Ireland, we are facing an increasing shortage of nurses, a shortage which is being filled by foreign nurses who are being induced to come here, even though the nursing shortage may be as bad or worse in their own countries. Is the substantial drop-out of Irish nurses in training and of qualified nurses working in hospitals caused by economic, social or cultural factors, or is it related to a decline in the attributes of caring and compassion which appeared to motivate people more in former, less privileged times? It is obviously related among other causes to the wider career choices available to nurses nowadays.

Perhaps the major cause of the current decline in the numbers of Irish nurses in our hospitals can be attributed to the loss of our hospital nursing schools and the more technical training of young nurses for their first three or four years on the university campus since 2002. While the number of applicants for nursing remains at a satisfactory level, there is now a huge clinical drop-out among undergraduates and postgraduates, a phenomenon which was not a problem in the days of the hospital school. It would be worth enquiring whether the same shortage pertained in other Western countries at the time they adopted the university training system. Is the candidate for nursing who spends the first three or four years mostly on the university campus likely to retain the full flush of enthusiasm and compassion for the sick which often lie behind the choice of nursing in the first place? Poor financial rewards and irregular hours are often cited as problems in attracting people to the nursing profession, but I would question these assumptions. In earlier years, these considerations appeared to have little influence on a profession which was traditionally dedicated to patient care, and nowadays the conditions of nursing have been greatly improved.

Those of us specialists who had dedicated hospital departments were fortunate that there was little change in the nursing staff over time. Agency nurses were unknown, and many staff nurses and most ward sisters remained in the same hospital for many years and became valued members of the institution.

It is right that nurses should have a third-level education at the university level and that they should be granted an undergraduate degree of the same standing as other graduates. But surely a greater proportion of their undergraduate years should be spent on the hospital campus, in direct contact with patients and acquiring experience of patient care. Having acquired their basic nursing degree, they can then specialise, as is the custom in the medical profession.

In my own experience, the first three years on the university campus learning the basic sciences was excessively long and probably not as productive for a young, active mind as it should have been. This part of the training could quite easily have been compressed into two years or less. It lacked any stimulus for young people preparing to enter a caring profession. One hundred and twenty callow youths and twenty diffident young women, and a distant contact with faculty members, made for little inspiration and made a mockery of the claim to the Newman tradition of a university. As an undergraduate, all changed as I spent the last three of my six years in the hospital with relatively little time attending lectures in the university. My time in the hospital was not only a vital contribution to my clinical training but was inspirational in the vocational context and left me with a lifetime interest in my profession and in my teaching hospital. My first three years in the university gave me little inkling of the pride I was to take in my future profession. If nurses in training spent more time on the hospital campus, their commitment to nursing and their loyalty to their own teaching hospital would be enhanced, to the benefit of both the institution and patients.

In one publication, Madeline Spiers, the current president of the Irish Nurses' Organization, underlines the difficulties under which nurses and midwives have to work, and attributes much of their problems to health-service policies which are driven by bureaucrats, with little input from health professionals, who are nearer the coal-face.[44] In particular, she attributes the excessive workload of nurses and the abnormally high ratio of patients to nurses in Ireland to the fact that the nursing profession at the clinical level is not consulted about problems about which the nurses are best informed. She goes on to say:

> The difficulties arising from overcrowding, such as increased cross-infection, loss of privacy and dignity, increased waiting times for treatment, all negatively impact upon patient care. It is trite to suggest, as the minister has, that 'you do not need money to wash your hands'. The constant objective, in recent years, has been developing management systems and not enhanced patient care. There has been no support for the nurse or midwife who was concerned about the lowering of standards of care.

It is impossible for a physician of my vintage, however much I concede the reality and inevitability of change, not to look back with nostalgia to the days when we had our own nursing school, when our nurses remained for many years in the service of the hospital, when they remained friends of the hospital all their lives, and when we never heard of agency nurses. These may be sentimental ramblings, but we can still retrieve some of the better aspects of past days by providing nurses in training with more time and more practical work on the hospital campus and with a closer tie to their chosen hospital. These suggestions might ruffle the feathers of the faculty members in the universities, but the current establishment responsible for nurses' training should be flexible in deciding policy and should be prepared to learn from the past when planning for the future.

The nursing profession is inseparable from the medical profession in terms of ethos, professional calling and dedication to patient care.

5

THE ROLE OF GOVERNMENT

On the 10 April 2006, the *Irish Medical News* published a short summary of the future health policies of the political parties coming up to the general election, scheduled for early 2007. The Fianna Fáil policy shows how electoral considerations will lead to a sense of unreality because political parties are primarily interested in their own political success. The recent Fianna Fáil policy statement commences with a summary of its future objectives for health if returned to government:

> The development of a world-class public health service; a combination of greater investment and a reform of the system will provide a high-quality and accessible health service for all. It will ensure a major expansion in the level and quality of services throughout the country and *it will ensure the end of a two-tier healthcare system* by ensuring that public patients will have access to timely and quality services in all parts of the system. [Italics added.]

These aspirations are shared to varying degrees by the other parties in parliament. The electorate is entitled to feel a little sceptical about such rosy promises in the light of previous failed undertakings but, more cogently, the electorate is entitled to ask that health be removed from politics and that future health policies be decided by an all-party group in consultation with appropriate advisors in the health and public domain. Why, if the present government intends to adopt a one-tier system – reflecting the view of some of the opposition parties – has it made no attempt to do so during its long time in government? It is hard to be convinced of the government's sincerity in undertaking this long-term objective. Ms Harney's philosophy of health conforms to the development of an increasingly divisive two-tier system, and the Taoiseach and his party must be perfectly aware of this. I suspect that the author of the government's future policies on health was hardly aware of the problems which exist in health care and of the failings of social justice in this country.

The situation is further confused by a statement made by Mary Harney when she was attending the Whitfield Clinic in Waterford:

> The HSE has my full support in procuring quality services for patients from private not-for-profit independent providers or from the public sector.[45]

Up to now, the option of either a one- or two-tier system has been one of the more contentious areas among the political groups, and the government's recently announced commitment to a one-tier system must come as a surprise. I suspect that there is no basic plan established by government, and perhaps by any political party, to cope with our mounting medical and related social problems. And to compound the problems of providing an optimal health service, there is little contact and less mutual understanding between the medical professions and the government, as represented by the minister, Ms Harney.

It is extraordinary that the government is implementing health policies of a fundamental and contentious nature without any public or professional consultation or debate, and that current policies will entrench a highly inequitable two-tier system which will land us inexorably with the problems inherent in the American system of health care. One might expect that, in order to achieve an optimal health service in the current confused circumstances, we would require comprehensive research into other national systems and wide consultation with doctors, economists, insurers and the public, as well as with parliament and the political parties. Instead, over the years, we have been subjected to various hasty and ill-judged decisions, with no long-term planning of a comprehensive system of health care, and apparently little attention to the basic recommendations of the various commissions set up by the Departments of Health and Finance in recent years.

In *Unhealthy State: The Anatomy of a Sick Society*, Ms Wren states that 'the political system is one of the barriers to reform, if not the major one' (page 84). The government, and the role of politicians, are dealt with in great detail by Ms Wren. She might have added the confused central policies of successive government over the years, with executive indecision in the face of different minority pressure groups. It is clear that, from the end of World War II, successive Irish governments have failed to establish a coherent and rational policy in relation to the health services. The want of good government in this area may be excused, bearing in mind the failure to predict the rapid advances in medical care and technology, the rampant cost of such advances, the increasing expectations of a better educated and more litigious public, and a service which is doctor-led. Nevertheless, most other Western countries have shown better vision in adapting to the social, demographic and health changes over the past fifty years.

It is reasonable to claim that the Irish system has evolved in a piecemeal manner, with little co-ordinated central planning, and with government's failure to impose its policies because of dissenting and minority groups, local politicians and local loyalties conflicting with national exigencies, and a profession which is conservative with regard to radical changes in our health-care system. Brennan, in her report, refers to the Department of Health's fragmented record, and she is particularly critical of the civil servants' lack of accountability. Unfortunately, in every single aspect of the health services the Brennan report examined, low standards of accountability, and a complacent and casual attitude in this respect from the public servants in charge of taxpayers' money, were found.

One might attribute government failures to conceive and impose well-planned policies on our particular brand of the party system, where there is a trend by government to put party and electoral considerations before responsibilities to the community. Ms Wren refers repeatedly to the government's supine response to the minority groups who successfully resist efforts to bring about necessary changes in the health-delivery service. She reminds us how generally ineffective the Department of Health has been since it was established in 1946.

Both David Lloyd George and Winston Churchill, in their separate musings about democracy, universal suffrage and the parliamentary system, had reservations about the party system. Lloyd George wrote about the evils of the party structure in parliament and looked with disfavour on party control.[46] This view receives support when, in situations of emergency such as war, coalition governments are formed to eliminate the influence of narrow party interests.

We can certainly share the same view about the current situation in Ireland. Every aspect of public life, and every branch of administration, including health, education, transport and local government, to mention a few, has suffered because of the failure of our democratically elected leaders to put the public good before their determination to remain in power. The Platonic concept of democratic leadership, based on integrity and detachment from personal gain, which we enjoyed in Ireland from the foundation of the State until the 1950s, is a thing of the past and can be retrieved only through radical changes in public ethics and in the electoral system which prevails in Ireland. The only leader in our eighty-four-year history as an independent country who did not favour control of government by party was William T. Cosgrave. He refused the leadership of the Cumann na nGaedheal Party in the early 1920s because he believed that the country's political leader should be above the influence of party politics.

Winston Churchill was less than enthusiastic about the political system in the United Kingdom in the 1920s, believing that it no longer attracted the ablest people in government.[47] Can we attract the ablest and most trustworthy ministers in Ireland under our party and electoral system, bearing in mind the financial opportunities available to talented and educated people in business and in the professions, the hassles involved in politics, and the uncertainties of a political life?

Desirable changes might be achieved by the elimination of the rigid whip system in parliament (except perhaps for a limited number of finance bills) and by the creation of single-seat constituencies with the transferrable vote to allow our TDs to devote their time, energies and skills to central affairs, and not to be constantly looking over their shoulders to constituency affairs and electoral rivals from the same party who may be beavering away locally to attract the favour of their constituents. We should reduce the number of TDs, pay them better (at least as well as medical consultants or high court judges), and welcome the recent dual mandate legislation, which prevents TDs from membership of local councils and committees, where political privilege can be abused. The one-seat system would ease the concern of the elected representative in the Dáil about local affairs and might eliminate many of the local obstacles to national progress.

Where central government has been most at fault is in its failure to provide for the adequate needs of the old, the lonely and the disabled, despite our recent prosperity. Many patients who occupy beds in the Dublin hospitals are there because they are awaiting discharge to more suitable institutions or to their homes, where no assistance may be available to care for them. And not a few are in hospital awaiting transport or the support of relatives. It must be clear that, if we had more efficient means of discharging patients, this would make a significant difference to our exceptionally long waiting lists – the main reason for the inequalities in our health-delivery system.

Government in recent years in Ireland has certainly failed to give the principled and ethically led leadership which ensures the welfare of society. It has failed to provide the accountability which is required to ensure responsible citizenship and, by its own example, has even contributed to tarnishing the principles of the electorate in that it has failed to control corporate and personal corruption. This failure, whether cause or effect, may well be symptomatic of an increasingly corrupt society. Government is at a disadvantage, in the context of individual rights and of an intrusive and influential media, in trying to solve as complex a problem as our health service in view of the mounting social, professional and political problems already alluded to, and of the many dissident, vocal and influential groups who may, for personal reasons, wish to hinder a cohesive and constructive solution to the nation's health structure. Nor are the policies of our current health minister, with her knee-jerk innovations, consistent with good government. They may be expedient in the short term but can only be disastrous in achieving a long-term equitable system of health care.

Because of the degree of personal freedom which prevails and is so highly valued in our country (without necessarily a corresponding degree of personal responsibility to the community), the commitment to democracy may suffer or indeed may contain the seeds of its own destruction. Parliament in Ireland appears to be losing out to other influences, such the lobbying constituency which operates directly through the ministers without consultation with Dáil Éireann, just as essentially political matters may be decided by media pressure or the law courts rather than by the people through parliament.

Ireland's phenomenal advance in prosperity during the last two decades provided a huge opportunity to expand our social services and to narrow the divide between rich and poor. However, we have not taken advantage of our good fortune: much of this prosperity has been squandered on cars, holidays, holiday homes and amassing wealth, in a culture of excess, the problems of which are compounded by the political parties' almost obsessional commitment to maintaining a low-tax regime.

According to a recent poll reported by RTÉ, the first two choices of those who are about to receive their SSIA funds are a new car and a Continental holiday! A less selfish public policy, with higher taxes devoted to righting the problems which are endemic in health care, education, public transport and the environment, and with enlightened legal and political reform, would have provided a shining light to the world of what a modern democracy can do to celebrate material prosperity. It is likely that Mary Harney's intention to keep taxes low – a policy loudly proclaimed at the PDs' annual conference on 22 April 2006 and at the Fianna Fáil Ard Fheis in November 2006 – was likely to appeal to the electorate at the next election rather than to those who would wish to see a more equitable, safer, better educated and more environmentally responsible society.

Now that we are faced with an obesity syndrome of epidemic proportions, which we share with other Western countries, we can only deplore the lack of an effective policy to encourage all ages to become more aerobically active, particularly during leisure hours. Successive governments, and virtually all local authorities, have neglected to implement a comprehensive programme to encourage cycling and walking in our cities, towns and countryside. Hundreds of housing estates, big and small, are constructed without safe and adequate cycling facilities for children and adults, as recommended more than ten year ago by the Commission on Cycling organised by John Gormley TD when he was Lord Mayor of Dublin. Adding well-designed cycle tracks would cost little, at least compared to the cost of roads, and better facilities for walking and sport for young and old would probably cost society nothing because of the associated savings in energy consumption, as well as reduced crime and vandalism. Legislation and effective education on the nutritional needs of a society are also awaited by those concerned about the advance of the obesity syndrome.

We have many non-governmental organisations (NGOs) established to encourage health promotion and to support specific groups of patients. While there is increasing rapport between the NGOs and the Department of Health and other government agencies, the NGOs should be encouraged to maintain and increase their role in the health services with the support of government and the Health Services Executive.

In the past, the army and the Garda were noted for their involvement in sport and athletics. The Garda were noted for their vibrant boxing club, which had a national and international reputation in the boxing world. They also had a successful rowing club and a programme of athletics and physical training. The army was also noted for its athletic prowess. Most competitive sport seems to have lapsed in both forces, although in the army the men must undergo a physical fitness examination annually. The men of the two forces are no longer the icons of the public as they were formerly. One Garda informant told me that double-jobbing left little time for the men to enjoy competitive sport!

We also face the serious problem of the rapid growth in the

number of SUVs ferrying children to school, with serious effects in terms of cost, the environment, public health and community life. We can tolerate ministers who propose to spend €32 billion on a public-transport system to cope with the burgeoning car population, whereas there is no mention made of the bicycle, and not enough of the need for better public transport.

Our meteoric change from modest circumstances to wealth has had undesirable effects of greed and waste, which contrasts with our more modest and generous spirit of the past. Our obsession with material things and with self-gratification clouds our insight into the long-term psychological and environmental consequences of our worldly culture. It has to be said that the performance of recent administrations during the Celtic Tiger leaves much to be desired in the areas of social and health-prevention legislation. The minister for state in the Department of Health and Children, Mr Seán Power, speaking at a Senate debate about the long-awaited Men's National Health Policy, had this to say:

> A great challenge in the years ahead is perhaps the need to strengthen the evidence base on men's health in Ireland and identify what works best in different contexts.

I expect he was referring primarily to men's exercise, drinking and smoking habits, and nutrition. We look forward to Mr Power's early initiative to improve the health of men, but he will only succeed if he follows the radicalism of his colleague Micheál Martin. Can Mr Power resist the current trends towards more sedentary activity and obesity in the population and provide the facilities for everyone to take adequate aerobic exercise? At least we can give deserved credit to Minister Martin and the government after the smoking legislation.

6

Health Promotion

Our health service has to be a misnomer: a disproportionate amount of the cost is devoted to treating sick people and only a small fraction to health promotion. To the public at large, medical care implies better health, but our current health service is not designed to improve health. We doctors reduce morbidity and mortality, but we often add little to positive health or longevity. Better education of all classes will bring far greater rewards in terms of health and longevity than the 'ideal' health system, whatever that may be. In the light of the rapidly increasing cost of caring for the sick and the disabled, and of occasional failures in clinical judgement, it is unlikely that we shall ever provide a sickness service which will satisfy both client and provider, particularly as some relatives and colleagues view death as abnormal and life to be extended at all costs.

It is now apparent that, with our knowledge of the causes of chronic diseases, and in the favourable ambience of Western countries today, more and more people are living close to the full human life-span of a hundred years without suffering much more than an occasional upper-respiratory-tract infection. Whatever about the rare genetic diseases, the last two or three decades, with the dramatic declines in heart disease, stroke, lung cancer and respiratory disease, have taught us that, more than anything else, bringing about changes in personal behaviour must be the principal objective of a health service. The 'ideal' health system is an illusion based on a burgeoning drug culture and a belief that doctors can provide a cure for all our ills. With increasing technology and an ever-more-demanding public, health services are threatening to become a bottomless pit in terms of cost, and many forms of treatment are of doubtful cost efficacy.

If medical care is equivalent to health care, then social and preventive medicine must assume its full responsibility for the health of the community. It cannot abrogate this responsibility to the present system of health care. If by 'medical care' is meant a coping with the existing state of ill-health, without attempting to effect changes in human behaviour, then we have a state of stagnation which can only lead to failure with regard to health improvement. We need better training and a greater allocation of doctors, nurses and social scientists in the preventive services. We should also be vigorously attacking current social problems of importance, including alcoholism, poor nutrition, violence, the destruction of the environment, lack of physical exercise, and diminishing social cohesion. Perhaps we should also seek to engender a better philosophy of rationality and spirituality in order to counter the dedication to power, possessions and money which is consuming Western society and is endangering the Earth and humanity.

At various points, Wren refers to the neglect of health promotion and the need for more emphasis on health education. It is hardly necessary to note the poor constituency that preventive medicine has within the profession and among our politicians. Any mention of health promotion is still received by many doctors and politicians with a glazed look, although in recent years there has been more emphasis on the promotion of health and personal responsibility for health. This trend is already showing benefit in terms of falling levels of the chronic non-communicable diseases and of increasing life expectancy for both men and women.

If we were to become an active, health-promoting society, it is difficult to assess the likely effect on the cost of the health service. One might think that there would be a marked increase in the cost of caring for the aged sick and infirm. However, there is little doubt that a cultural shift towards personal responsibility for health would lead to a greatly improved life expectancy and should reduce the period of chronic disability and loss of independence which is a feature in our ageing population and which makes the care of the elderly so expensive for society. This view is supported by many research papers which find a significant improvement in the physical and psycho-social health, and a shorter period of disability, in older people, which parallels the increasing longevity in the Western World.[48, 49]

The seeds of chronic illness, of repeated hospitalisation, and of loss of independence in older people are most frequently sown in middle age, when unhealthy lifestyles lead to the emergence of self-induced disease. In a perfect world, we should anticipate living a normal life-span and remaining independent of others and of our medical services until we are close to the end of our days. An optimum sickness service on its own will not provide us with a perfect world.

Some of our medical and surgical colleagues will attribute the improved life expectancy to advances in medical and surgical intervention, but the evidence confirms beyond doubt that the identification of the causes of the chronic diseases since World War II and the adoption of healthier lifestyles based on this evidence, particularly among the better educated, accounts for the major advances that have been made in health and longevity in recent years.

In my own sphere of cardiology, there can be little doubt about the dominant role of prevention in the achievement of a healthy society. Thanks largely to preventive measures in relation to smoking, healthy eating and blood-pressure control, the coronary epidemic, which peaked in the late nineteen sixties and early nineteen seventies in England and Wales, has shown a dramatic mortality decline, of about 62 percent in men and 45 percent in women. The decline is most evident in the younger age groups. This led to an estimated saving of 68,230 deaths in 2000. Such a finding is confirmed in a study by Unal and his colleagues,[50] who attributed 48 percent of the decline to reduced cigarette smoking, 9.5 percent to hypertension control, and 9.5 percent to lowered cholesterol levels – obviously the result of healthier eating. Forty-two percent of the decline in coronary mortality was attributed by Unal and his colleagues to treatment including secondary prevention, treatment of heart failure, and treatment of acute myocardial infarction. Only 3.5 percent was attributed to heart surgery and angioplasty combined. Small adverse effects were attributed to reduced exercise, increasing obesity, and diabetes. The population reduction in hypertension in Britain was attributed in another study to lifestyle change rather than medication.[51]

In Ireland, the decline in mortality from coronary heart disease is similar to that in Britain. A study from St James's Hospital in Dublin reports the same findings among the Irish population, where the decline was 47 percent between 1985 and 2000, with an estimated saving of 3,800 lives.[52] Again, 48 percent of the decline was attributed to a sharp fall in cigarette smoking among the middle-aged. The decline in heart disease is common to all Western countries and shows a gradual convergence, as is evident from Figure 2.

FIGURE 2: Age-standardised death rates per 100,000 population from coronary heart disease, men 1968–99, selected countries (Source: WHO)

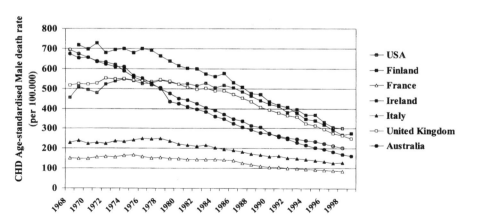

*Coronary Heart Disease: ICD codes 410-414 (8th and 9th revision), I20-I25

The dominant influence of lifestyle in reducing coronary mortality has been confirmed in the United States, where between 1980 and 1990 57 percent of the reduction was attributed to risk-factor intervention;[53] in New Zealand, where between 1982 and 1993 52 percent of the reduction was attributed to risk-factor intervention;[54] and in Scotland, where 60 percent of the reduction from 1975 and 1994 was attributed to the same cause.[55] There is little doubt that treatment of the established disease has improved during these two decades, but lifestyle changes are also being adopted more widely. Such changes have made by far the greatest contribution to the decline – and at a fraction of the cost to society. There is little doubt that heart surgery and angioplasty have limited value in the management of patients with chronic coronary disease.

It is no longer acceptable that the medical profession pay little attention to health promotion. Although it is understandable that in the past, when little was known about the causes of our common chronic non-communicable diseases, doctors had little opportunity to advise the public about the avoidance of heart disease, stroke and respiratory disease. Today, thanks largely to the dedicated work of the medical epidemiologists, we have extensive knowledge about causation. With the authority we wield with our patients and the public, we can have a profound effect on public health if we practice preventive medicine in tandem with our traditional role as doctors. For reasons of training, and a long tradition of caring for the sick, it is understandable that doctors are more attracted to interventional medicine than to health promotion, and that they are more concerned with managing symptoms rather than causes. This is also understandable because of the advantages we clinicians have financially, and the close and influential contact we have with our patients.

There are undoubtedly huge opportunities for improving the health of the middle-aged and older population through a cultural change in society aimed at adopting responsibility for one's own health and that of one's family, and by regulating the imbalance between the sickness service and the promotion of good health. Public education and public example are the key to better health in the community: the better-educated in Ireland and Britain have a substantially better health record than those with less education, almost certainly because the better-educated are more responsive to the health message. The mortality of Social Class 3 in Britain is three times greater at the age of sixty compared to the more educated Social Class 1. I expect that the same disparity exists in the Republic and in the North. Research carried out by the Institute of Public Health (IPH) shows that mortality rates among the poor in Ireland are 100 to 200 percent higher than among the rich. The director of the IPH, Dr Jane Wilde, said that political leadership and policy coherence are essential in order to tackle the wide gap between rich and poor in this country.[56]

The Health Promoting Hospitals movement, which started in Ireland and Europe in the mid-1980s, holds out considerable hope that the health professions will take a more proactive part in health promotion and in public education on health and related matters. Hospitals, while founded to look after the sick, can by virtue of their ethos and their role in the community have a profound effect on health promotion through direct contact with patients and their relatives, and with the wider public. The hospital's increasing involvement in rehabilitation and secondary prevention is providing an important link between its services to the sick and the preventive measures which are emerging as a direct result of the research into the causes of the common chronic diseases. In my own alma mater, St Vincent's University Hospital, a department of preventive medicine and health promotion has been in existence for thirty years.[57] It was an early innovation and has made an important contribution to the hospital as an institution with a holistic commitment to the health of the community. Every large teaching hospital should have a department of health promotion and prevention, in tandem with the more academic departments of health promotion and epidemiology in the associated universities.

Ms Wren is wrong in assuming that life expectancy depends on a nation's wealth and a good health service. On page 240, she writes:

> Only when all citizens can access adequately resourced primary care and when hospitals treat the most ill first can Irish life expectancy and health be expected to improve significantly relative to other EU states.

She disagrees with the minister of state at the Department of Health in 1999, Frank Fahy, who was concerned about healthy lifestyles within the service, while she appears to approve of the chief medical officer in the Department of Health, Dr Jim Kiely, when he said that health was related to the problem of inequitable access to health services based on need.

Good medical facilities may play a small part in improving life expectancy, but the lifestyle of the population, and a proactive approach from government in encouraging exercise, non-elitist sport, healthy nutrition and moderation in alcohol consumption are much more important. Above all, good government must ensure that every citizen is provided with the very best educational opportunities. Doctors can treat the sick and help the disabled, but our role in extending life is limited compared to the potential of health education and the influence of good governance.

REFERENCES

ABBREVIATIONS

BMJ	British Medical Journal
IMJ	Irish Medical Journal
IMN	Irish Medical News
IMT	Irish Medical Times
JAMA	Journal of the Americal Medical Association
JRCP	Journal of the Royal College of Physicians
MW	Medicine Weekly
RCPI	Royal College of Physicians in Ireland

1. Barrington, Ruth, *Health, Medicine and Politics in Ireland, 1900–1970* (Institute of Public Administration, 1987), 348
2. Tussing, A. D. and M.-A. Wren, *How Ireland Cares: The Case for Health Reform* (New Ireland, Dublin, 2006), 434
3. Feachem, R. G. A., K. S. Neelan and L.W. Karen, 'Earning more for their dollar: A comparison of the National Health Service with California's Kaiser Permanente', *BMJ* 2002; 324, 135–41
4. 'A Discussion Document on the Feasibility of a Compulsory Specialist and Hospital Insurance Scheme as an Alternative to the Present Irish System', *IMJ* 1975; 68, suppl. pp1–4, editorial p577
5. Wren, Maev-Ann, *Unhealthy State: Anatomy of a Sick Society* (New Island, Dublin, 2003), 445
6. Barrett, A. and A. Bergin, 'Assessing Age-related Pressures on the Public Finances, 2005–2050' (ESRI, 2005)
7. *MW*, 8/3/06
8. *Irish Times*, 21/3/06
9. *IMN*, 24/4/06
10. *MW*, 29/3/06
11. *MW*, 22/2/06
12. *IMT*, 27/3/06
13. Mulcahy, R. 'Are we practising evidence-based cardiology?', *IMJ* 2006; 99, 37–9

14 *IMT*, March 2006
15 *IMN*, 18/7/05
16 *Wall Street Journal*, 30/5/97
17 *BMJ*, 2006; 333, 57
18 Touhy C. H., C. M. Flood and M. J. Stabile, 'How does private finance affect public health care systems? Marshalling the evidence from OECD countries', *Health Politics, Policy and Law*, 2004; 29, 359–96
19 *IMT*, 31/3/06
20 *BMJ*, 2006; 333, 59
21 Mitchell, D., '25 Years: An Interim History of the Royal College of Physicians of Ireland 1963–1988' (RCPI, 1992)
22 Hunter, Ian (ed.), 'Cheering up the patient' (Goodbody Stockbrokers, 2005)
23 *Irish Times*, 1/11/05
24 *MW*, March 2006
25 *IMN*, 23/3/06
26 *MW*, 12/4/06
27 *IMN*, 25/4/06
28 *IMT*, 31/3/06
29 *Irish Times* Health Supplement, 1/11/05
30 *MW*, 31/5/06
31 *IMN*, 29/10/05
32 *Irish Times*, 28/9/05
33 *MW*, 23/3/06
34 *MW*, 8/3/06
35 *MW*, 10/5/06
36 Garcia, M. J., J. Lessick and M. H. Hoffmann, 'Computed Tomography for Assessment of Coronary Artery Stenosis', *JAMA* 2006; 296, 403–11
37 O'Sullivan, J. J., P. Leavey and R. Mulcahy, 'Inappropriate long-term medication in patients admitted to a coronary care unit', *JRCP*, 1989; 23, 232–5
38 *IMN*, 27/3/06
39 *Irish Times* Health Supplement, 7/3/06
40 *IMT*, 17/3/06
41 'First Report of the Joint Working Party on the Organisation of Medical Work in Hospitals' (H.M. Stationery Office, 1967)
42 Nelson, Bataldam et al., 'Microsystems in Health Care', *Journal on Quality Improvement*, Sept 2002 to Nov 2003; vols 2, 3
43 *IMT*, March 2006
44 *Irish Times*, 16/3/06
45 *IMN*, 8/11/06
46 Owen, Frank, *Tempestuous Journey – Lloyd George: His Life and Times* (Hutchinson, 1954)

47 Churchill, Winston, *Thoughts and Adventures* (Odhams Press, London, 1932)
48 Baltcs, P. B. and K. V. Mayer (eds), *The Berlin Ageing Study*, Cambridge University Press, 1999
49 Rowe, J. W. and R. L. Kahn, *Successful Ageing* (Pantheon Books, New York, 1998)
50 Unal, B., J. A. Critchly and S. Capewell, 'Explaining the Decline in Coronary Heart Disease Mortality in England and Wales Between 1981 and 2000', *Circulation*, 2004; 109, 1101–7
51 Tunstall, Pedoe et al., 'Patterns of Declining Blood Pressure Across Replicate Surveys of the WHO Monica Project, Mid-1980s to Mid-1990s, and the Role of Medication', *BMJ* 2006; 332, 629
52 Bennett K, et al. 'Explaining the recent decrease in coronary heart disease mortality rates in Ireland', *Journal of Epidemiology and Community Health*, 2006; 60, 322–27
53 Hunink, M. G., L. Goldman, A. N. Tostesen et al., 'The recent decline in mortality from coronary heart disease, 1980–1990: The effect of secular trends in risk factor and treatment,' *JAMA*, 1997; 277, 535–42
54 Capewell S., R. Beaglehole, M. Seddon et al., 'Explaining the decline in coronary heart disease mortality in Auckland, New Zealand between 1982 and 1993', *Circulation* 2000; 102ff, 1511–16
55 Capewell S., C. E. Morrison and J. J. McMurray, 'Contribution of modern cardiovascular treatment and risk-factor changes to the decline in coronary heart disease mortality in Scotland between 1975 and 1974', *Heart*, 1999; 81, 380–86
56 *IMN*, 23/10/06
57 Mulcahy, R., 'The Department of Preventive Medicine and Health Promotion at St Vincent's University Hospital', *MW*, 6/2/06

Glossary of Medical Terms

Angina Can be chronic or unstable angina. The pain in chronic angina tends to be constant in severity and is generally induced by exercise or stress.

Angiogram An X-ray showing the inside of arteries by injecting opaque dye through a fine tube or catheter inserted into a leg or arm artery.

Angioplasty Involves a fine tube with an inflatable balloon at its tip being inserted into a coronary artery to distend a blockage.

Atherosclerosis A cholesterol-rich deposit found in many arteries of the body. It is most evident in the arteries supplying the heart, brain, aorta and leg vessels and causes obstructions and clotting in these vessels.

CAT scan Computer-assisted tomography, an advanced form of X-ray.

Coronary artery One of the two main arteries which supply the heart with blood.

Coronary heart disease Present where there is clinical or ECG evidence of coronary artery disease because of a heart attack, angina or other heart symptoms.

ECG A recording of the electrical activity which controls the heart muscle function.

Endothelium The delicate lining of an artery, which prevents clotting in the healthy vessel. When damaged, or if it becomes unstable for any reason, clots may form in the vessel.

Heart attack Refers to any form of sudden heart disturbance. It is most often used to describe a myocardial infarction or acute angina.

Heart surgery Coronary surgery aims to attach new blood vessels in order to bypass blockages.

MRI Magnetic resonance imaging. A non-radiation form of imaging of the tissues

Myocardial infarction The common form of heart attack. It refers to the heart damage which occurs when the blood supply to part of the heart muscle may be reduced or cut off.

Stenosis A partial or complete blockage in an artery.

Stent A short metal or plastic tube which is inserted during angioplasty to maintain the patency of an opened blockage.

Stress test Refers to the performance of the ECG during exercise to reveal changes which may not be evident in the conventional ECG performed at rest.

Stroke Any disturbance of brain function leading to paralysis or other abnormalities of mental or physical function. It is generally caused by blockage in one of the carotid arteries or their main branches, or by brain haemorrhage caused by high blood pressure, an aneurysm in the brain, or an accident.